Lectin Free

Cookbook

300 Everyday Recipes for Beginners and Advanced Users.
Try Easy and Healthy Lectin Free Recipes

Copyright © 2019

All Rights Reserved.

By Markus Olsen

Table of contents

4

Vegetarian Recipes

Salad and Sides Recipes

Introduction

Chapter 1

Since life has started on Earth, each day something new is happening. There are advancements in every field of life that came out as man learnt how to live. Initially, there was no difference between a man and an animal but as time proceeded, he came to know who is he and what his purpose of living is. Man learned that he is different from animals. He got knowledge which revealed the truth of life on him. Early man was a hunter of food. He did not have the sense that what is good for him and what is not. Not even he knew that whether the things he is hunting to eat are for him to eat, or not.

But today the world is developed enough to understand things that favor the human race. Food is necessary for the life of a human. If we do not eat, we would die. Now it's not only important to eat but, eat what is good for you. It is necessary to make a good choice for your food because whatever you select to eat affects your today and tomorrow. Good food and nutrition are important if you want to live a healthy lifestyle.

Chapter 2
Understanding the lectin free diet

Lectins that pose a danger for humans are the following two i.e. prolamins and agglutinins. Those lectins which are having a higher quantity of amino acids are called prolamins like gluten etc. while the example of agglutininsare kidney beans etc. The following will help you understand lectins better.

What are lectins?

So, what actually are lectins? Lectins are the naturally occurring proteins. These proteins are found in the food we eat. Lectins are mostly found in grains, legumes, seeds that we eat. Apart from this some vegetables also contain lectins. In a little amount, we can find lectins in our dairy products. Lectins that we eat help our body in its proper functioning. And how this happens is that those lectins help cells to communicate and interact with each other. We can find lectins commonly in the food we eat. We eat wheat, potatoes, beans, seeds, and, tomatoes that contain lectins.

If we go back in time or if we just take our minds to the time when life started, there were no animals. First plants were here and animals came after them. Plants were all happy and the first to inhabit earth but as time proceeded animals came to existence. Now plants were not able to live freely and all their independent existence was under a heavy burden. First plants did not have any danger because nobody was on Earth who could eat them, who could destroy them, who could dislocate them from where they live and build another house over there.

When animals did not come to earth there wasn't anyone who could create pollution and increase the difficulty for the life of plants. But as the animals gripped their living, plant race was much affected. So, there they decided to take the revenge! They decided to save themselves and generate such toxins that would fight against humans. So, these are lectins that are present in the food derived from a plant source. Lectin proteins are also found in almost all forms of life.

The proteins found in the foods such as plants, grains and beans are called lectins. They tend to bind with the carbohydrates which can help communicate the cells to interact with each other.

They are the proteins that cause inflammation and weight gain and they are found in plants. Lectins are found in many foods and they are ubiquitous in nature. Lectins maybe get disabled using some specific monosaccharide and oligosaccharides. They bind to ingest lectins from the grains, nightshade plants. They prevent them from binding with the carbohydrates and hence are useful for neutralizing lectins.

Lectins help out in interconnecting cells with other without the help of immune system. They are crucially important for joining the cell membranes together. Lectins that pose a danger for humans are the following two i.e. prolamins and agglutinins. Those lectins which are having a higher quantity of amino acids are called prolamins like gluten etc. while the example of agglutininsare kidney beans etc. The following will help you understand lectins better.

Lectins are made up of legumes and raw grains and are in that part of seed which transforms into leaves after growth. It is important to note that the quantity of lectin in food is uniform; however, due to different experimentations done by humans, the quantity today is different.

Lectins act as defense systems in plants against any microorganism threatening its wellbeing. Lectins consists of nitrogen which is essential for growth of plants. Lectins are not digested by human beings and they enter blood without any change. The best way to remove or lower the number of lectins in plants is by procedures which involve moist heating. Plant's starch efficiently reduces and converts to carbohydrates which are better for us as they are removed from the body effectively before causing harm. Some effective ways of removing lectins include peeling, deseeding, boiling, fermentation, sprouting, and pressure cooking and soaking. Detail of some of which is given below:

Fermentation

Fermentation involves allowing beneficial bacteria for the human body to grow which assists digestion and helps get rid of harmful substances. Many substances like natto, miso and tamari are used as fermented soy substances to allow fermentation. Fermentation allows vegetables like cabbage to become beneficial and carry lesser amount of anti-nutrients. People who have trouble eating grains have applied this process to treat grains and have found it beneficial for the removal of lectins. However, it is known that hard natured lectins are still unaffected even after fermentation. Thus, it may be best to avoid such foods all together or apply more than one method for the removal of lectins completely.

Sprouting

It is noticed that the number of lectins is reduced to a great extent in beans, grains and seeds after the process of sprouting. This process however, is more effective if applied over a longer period. It is also important to know that in certain rare cases the effect of lectins is seen to improve after sprouting (namely, in alfalfa). In this process, the coating of seeds is metabolized after germination which results in the removal of lectins.

Pressure cooking and Soaking

The important reason for boiling, rinsing and soaking of beans is to reduce the number of lectins which is done in every cuisine. This process is probably the most commonly applied and is known to be useful as well. Beans are soaked overnight and the water in them is changed from time to time to effectively remove lectins in them. In addition to this, baking soda is added to the water to remove lectins completely as it enhances this process.

However, despite everything, lectins can be beneficial too. A small quantity of lectins can help assist removal of bacteria from human digestive system. Research shows that lectins can help in diagnosing and identifying certain cancers. Studies are being done on the role of lectins in the defense mechanism and how lectins can help prevent bacteria, fungus and viruses from spreading in the human body and help reduce medical diseases.

Chapter 3
Importance of lectins for plants

The carbohydrate binding proteins possess importance for plants as well. Legume lectins are found in a smaller amount in seeds and belong to sugar-binding proteins. In plants, lectins would be present as legume lectins. Transgene studies were carried out which gave an idea that plant lectins are important for rhizobia binding. Rhizobia are bacteria that get fixed in the root nodules of legumes. The function of rhizobia is to fix nitrogen for the plants. Nitrogen-fixation is necessary to convert atmospheric nitrogen to a form that could become consumable. Nitrogen fixing bacteria are present in the root nodules of plants that fix nitrogen for those plants. Lectins are initially present in a bigger amount in plant seeds. As the plant grows the concentration of lectin decreases in the seeds. This is observed so from here a conclusion can be derived that lectins are important for plant seedlings in the process of germination. Germination can be said as the sprouting of a seedling from the seed that might be from angiosperms or gymnosperms. Germination is generally said as the process from which growth of an organism occurs, from a seedling or a similar structure. Lectins are not only important for germination of seeds but also for their survival.

Lectins and the medical research

Lectins are also important in the field of medicine and medical research. Blood in humans is divided into several types based on the presence of antigen and inherent characteristics. Glycoproteins and glycolipids might be present on the surface of red blood cells. Purified lectins can identify these so they perform a role in differentiation among blood groups. Dolichos is a genus of flowering plant that belongs to family Fabaceae. A lectin derived from Dolichos biflorus helps in the identification of those cells that belong to the A1 blood group. Ulex is commonly known as gorse, fuz or whin and belongs to a genus of flowering plant from Fabaceae. Ulex europaeus helps in identifying H blood group antigen. Vicia is a genus of about 140 species of flowering plants that are part of legume family Fabaceae. They are commonly called viches. N blood group is identified by Vicia graminea. Iberis is called as candytuft and belongs to family Brassicaceae. Iberis amara is used to identify M blood group antigen. Coconut milk contains lectin. A lectin derived from coconut milk helps in identifying Theros antigen. A lectin from genus Carex, that is the genus of grassy plants is used to identify R antigen. Lectins also favor the field of neuroscience. PHA-L is a lectin from kidney beans. Anterograde labeling method is a technique that is used to trace the path of efferent axons with PHA-L. Bananas Musa Acuminata and Musa Balbisiana give a lectin called as banlec. We get banlec as a predominant protein in the pulp of those bananas that are ripe. It can bind to mannose and oligosaccharide that contain mannose. A study was conducted in 2010 that showed banlec inhibits HIV replication. Achylectins have agglutinating activity against human A type erythrocytes. Anti-B agglutinins have an important role in research and routine blood grouping.

Lectins; as human enemies

Lectins are assisting the pathogens to kill humans. They are helping in biochemical warfare. Here most important and worth mentioning lectin that is fighting humans with its full zeal is ricin. Ricinus Communis is a highly toxic agent. Thus, carbohydrate binding protein is generated within the seeds of castor oil plant. If only a few grains are taken by a human that is like the size of table salt, that can kill human easily. The median lethal dose of ricin is 22 micro kilograms per kilogram of body weight. If ricin is taken through oral route, then some of its toxicity is reduced because it is deactivated in the stomach. According to an estimate 1 milligram of ricin per kilogram of body weight contributes to being a lethal dose. If ricin is taken through inhalation route or through an injection, then 1.78 milligrams of ricin could kill an adult. Ricin has two protein domains. A protein domain is a conserved part of a given protein sequence and tertiary structure that can generate the rest of the protein chain. The two domains of ricin include; the N-glycosidase that cleaves nucleobases from ribosomal RNA. This stops protein synthesis in a cell and eventually leads to death. The other domain includes the lectin that binds cell surface galactosyl residues and this enables the proteins to enter cells.

Lectins as biochemical tools

The chemical processes that occur in living organisms are referred to as biochemical and tools are those devices that assist us in our work making a task easier. Lectins are also being used as biochemical tools. Affinity chromatography involves the use of concanavalin A and other lectins that are available in the market. They are used in the process of purification of glycoproteins. A biochemical mixture can be separated by using affinity chromatography. This is based on the specific interactions that are present between antigens and antibodies, enzymes and substrates, receptors and ligands or proteins and nucleic acids. Glycoforms and carbohydrate structures are the basis on which proteins are characterized. Various methods that help in the characterization of proteins include blotting, affinity chromatography, affinity electrophoresis, affinity immunoelectrophoresis with lectins and, microarrays.

Lectins favor the study of atomic interactions

Lectins are also important in studying carbohydrate recognition that is further aided by proteins. PHA and concanavalin A, both are lectins that are derived from the legume family of plants. Proteins are recognized by carbohydrates and this process is assisted by these two lectins. They are widely used and are obtained easily. They are specific to types of sugars. Lectins that are leguminous have a crystalline structure. This characteristic helps to have a detailed insight into all types of atomic interactions. These atomic interactions would be between carbohydrates and proteins.

What is wrong with lectins

The lectins are hard to digest. They have an effect that they have the ability to overfeed certain species of gut bacteria and they can lead to gut dysbiosis. The gut dysbiosis is linked to variety of health conditions and are certainly not good for health.

They have an ability to interact with the gut barrier and can cause some serious damage to the cells that form the gut barrier or worse they can open up the junctions between the cells. Of course, the genetic susceptibility plays a big role that how your body reacts to this or what happens in your body. They are big contributors to the development of a leaky gut which is linked to a variety of health conditions.

Chapter 4
Foods to eat

According to the findings made by Dr. Gundry, following are the foods that are recommended and are considerably befitting for those individuals who are interested to control their lectin intake and limit the consumption of carbohydrates joining foods in an effective manner:

1. A-2 milk
2. Green and leafy vegetables
3. Cooked potatoes
4. Meats which are pasture rose
5. Onions
6. Garlic
7. Celery
8. Asparagus
9. Vegetables which are cruciferous in nature which are Brussels sprouts and Broccoli
10. Olives and extra virgin olive oil
11. Mushrooms

12. Avocado

Chapter 5
Foods to avoid

Apart from the foods that help to lower the levels of lectins in the body, there are also such foods which are high on the lectins and one should avoid eating them. According to the findings done by Dr. Gundry the following are the foods to avoid for the individuals who are looking forward to decrease the number of lectins in their body:

- Nightshade vegetables like peppers, potatoes, eggplants and tomatoes
- Legumes such as beans, lentils, peanuts
- Grain. If it is necessary to consume grains, though, better to use white flour rather than the whole wheat flour, as per Dr. Gundry's recommendation.
- Squash

Only in seasoned foods are allowed to be consumed otherwise the fruits as a whole are not recommended in lectin free diet plan.

Some foods have strictly not been recommended for the individuals who are looking forward to decrease their lectin level because these are high on the lectin and they will cause serious damage

- Corn
- Meats from the animals who are fed on corn
- A-1 milk

Lectins are those proteins that have the ability to bind to sugar molecules. Another name given to lectins is antinutrients. They are given this special kind of name because they decrease the ability of the body to absorb nutrients. As they are claimed to be natural defense agents of the plant, they trick animals to avoid plants in the diet as much they could. Lectin is present in many foods that is obtained from plant source or animal source. Even after this 30% of your food has it in a good amount. It's not possible to digest lectins by humans because our digestive system does not have this ability. They are passed out of the body as it is.

Chapter: 6
Tips for a Lectin-Free Diet

1. The best alternative for lectin free shopping is to visit online stores and wholesale clubs.
2. To make it cost effective, always divide your shopping list into sections and groups.
3. Always choose white grains over brown as brown grains have lectins in a large quantity.

4. It is recommended to peel all your fruits and remove the seeds before consuming.

5. Try to use a pressure cooker when on a lectin free diet.

6. If you consume foods which are natural in nature, it will be easier to drop lectins like extra virgin olive oil, green vegetables, olives and avocados etc.

Breakfast Recipes

Morning Mini-Bagels
Prep + Cook time: 15 minutes | Serves: 8-12

Nutritional Info (per serving)

Calories	_Fat (g)_	_Protein (g)_	_Carbs (g)_
284	11.1	6.1	40.7

Ingredients:

2 1/4 teaspoon sea salt

3 cups blanched almond flour

1 cup tapioca starch

2 teaspoons baking powder

2 tbs. monk fruit sweetener

2 tbs. white wine vinegar

1 pastured egg

Directions:

1. Let your oven preheat at 400 degrees F. Layer a baking sheet with wax paper.
2. Take a 10-inch pot and fill half of it with water. Boil it with quarter teaspoon salt.
3. Mix almond flour with remaining salt, baking powder, tapioca starch, and monk fruit.
4. Stir in half cup warm water along with vinegar. Mix well to form a smooth dough.
5. Make 12 small bagels out of this dough and keep them aside.

6. Add the bagels to remaining boiling water in three batches.
7. Transfer them to a plate after 1 minute of cooking using a slotted spoon.
8. Place the bagels in the baking sheet and brush them with whisked egg wash.
9. Bake them for about 10 minutes until turns golden.
10. Serve.

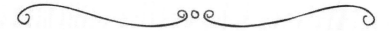

Warming Gingerbread
Prep + Cook time: 10 minutes | Serves: 1

Nutritional Info (per serving)

Calories	*Fat (g)*	*Protein (g)*	*Carbs (g)*
145	8.1	6.1	25.2

Ingredients:

1 tbs. almond butter, softened

1 tbs. coconut flour

1 tbs. cassava flour

1/2 teaspoon ground ginger

1/4 teaspoon cinnamon

pinch each of allspice, cloves, and nutmeg

1/2 teaspoon baking powder

2 teaspoons erythritol syrup

1/2 teaspoon apple cider vinegar

1/2 tbs. water

1 egg, lightly beaten

Directions:

1. Combine everything together in a microwave mug until it forms a smooth batter
2. Place this mug in the microwave for 1 and a half minute at high temperature.
3. Serve the muffin with cinnamon and melted butter on top.

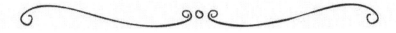

Cassava Flour Pancakes
Prep + Cook time: 15 minutes | Serves: 2-4

Nutritional Info (per serving)

Calories	Fat (g)	Protein (g)	Carbs (g)
161	8.4	3.4	22.9

Ingredients:

1 cup cassava flour

2 tbs. monk's fruit sweetener

1 tbs. baking powder

1 teaspoon cinnamon

1/4 teaspoon sea salt

1/8 teaspoon nutmeg

1 1/4 cup almond milk

1/2 teaspoon vanilla extract

2 large eggs room temperature

3 tbs. melted almond butter

1/4 cup water

Directions:

1. Place the griddled pan on medium-low heat.

2. Combine everything together in an electric mixer until it forms a smooth batter.
3. Pour ¼ cup of this batter into the hot griddled pan. Cook for it for 2 minutes per side.
4. Repeat the same step to make more pancakes.
5. Serve warm.

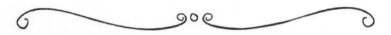

Vanilla Mug Muffin
Prep + Cook time: 10 minutes | Serves: 1

Nutritional Info (per serving)

Calories	Fat (g)	Protein (g)	Carbs (g)
341	17.4	4.1	45.3

Ingredients:

2 tbs. extra-virgin olive oil

1 tbs. coconut flour

1 tbs. cassava flour

2 teaspoons monk's fruit sweetener

1/2 teaspoon vanilla extract

1/2 teaspoon baking powder

pinch of sea salt

1 pastured egg, lightly beaten

a small handful of seasonal fruit or dark chocolate chips

Directions:

1. Combine everything together in a microwave mug until it forms a smooth batter
2. Place this mug in the microwave for 1 and a half minute at high temperature.

3. Serve the muffin with fruits or chocolate chips on top.

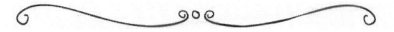

Peach Cobbler Pancake
Prep + Cook time: 15 minutes | Serves: 2

Nutritional Info (per serving)

Calories	Fat (g)	Protein (g)	Carbs (g)
197	8.1	6.1	25.2

Ingredients:

1 teaspoon vanilla essence

5 drops stevia liquid

5 ounces almond milk

1 tbs. coconut oil, melted

2 pastured eggs

1/4 teaspoon baking soda

1/4 cup coconut flour

1/4 teaspoon sea salt

1/4 cup tapioca flour

1/2 teaspoon baking powder

1/4 cup cassava flour

2 ripe peaches, peeled and sliced

cinnamon to garnish

Directions:

1. Combine everything together in an electric mixer starting with the wet ingredients then the dry ones.
2. Once the batter is smooth, then pour it into the pie pan.
3. Top it with peach slices and cinnamon ground.
4. Bake the pancake for 30 minutes.
5. Serve.

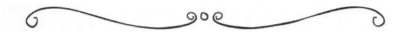

Egg, Spinach, and Cheese Burritos

Prep + Cook time: 15 minutes | Serves: 2-4

Nutritional Info (per serving)

Calories	*Fat (g)*	*Protein (g)*	*Carbs (g)*
288	23.7	17.5	2.1

Ingredients:

2 tbs.

extra-virgin olive oil

2 ounces spinach, chopped

2 cloves garlic, thinly sliced

Himalayan sea salt and black pepper

6 eggs, beaten

4 ounces goat cheese, crumbled

6-8-inch cassava flour tortillas

Directions:

1. Place a skillet on medium heat and stir in garlic, spinach, salt, and pepper.
2. Stir cook for 3 minutes then pour in eggs.
3. Scramble the egg after 30 seconds and cook for 4 minutes.
4. Spread the cheese over the egg.
5. Spoon this mixture into warmed tortillas.
6. Fold and serve.

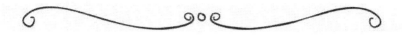

Vegan Pancakes

Prep + Cook time: 15 minutes | Serves: 2-4

Nutritional Info (per serving)

Calories	Fat (g)	Protein (g)	Carbs (g)
282	17.3	6.2	29.1

Ingredients:

1 cup almond flour

3/4 cup tapioca flour

1 Tbsp. baking powder

1/4 tsp. sea salt

2/3 cup unsweetened almond milk

2 tsp. apple cider vinegar

1 Tbsp. erythritol syrup

1 Tbsp. coconut oil, melted

1 tsp. pure vanilla extract

Directions:

1. Beat everything in a blender to get a smooth batter.
2. Place a greased skillet on medium heat.
3. Pour in ¼ cup of this batter into the skillet.
4. Cook for 2 minutes per side.
5. Make more pancakes using this way.
6. Serve with nut butter and vanilla sauce.
7. Enjoy.

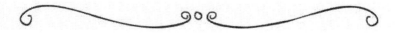

Sweet Potato Hash

Prep + Cook time: 30 minutes | Serves: 2-4

Nutritional Info (per serving)

Calories	Fat (g)	Protein (g)	Carbs (g)
309	14.5	2.8	44.4

Ingredients:

2 medium sweet potatoes, peeled and cubed

2 tbsp. olive oil or avocado oil

1 tsp. smoked paprika

½ tsp. turmeric

½ tsp. sea salt

½ tsp. onion powder

¼-1/2 Tsp. ground black pepper

2 cloves garlic, finely minced

Scallions, green parts only, sliced on a bias

Directions:

1. Let your oven preheat at 400 degrees F.
2. Toss sweet potatoes with oil, turmeric, salt, pepper, onion powder and paprika in a pan.
3. Spread them on a baking sheet. Roast them for 20 minutes.
4. Toss in garlic and return the pan to the oven for 5 minutes.
5. Garnish with scallions then serve

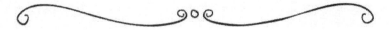

Broccoli Cheese Quiche
Prep + Cook time: 45 minutes | Serves: 4-6

Nutritional Info (per serving)

Calories	Fat (g)	Protein (g)	Carbs (g)
363	31.4	11.3	10.5

Ingredients:

Crust:

1/2 cup toasted macadamia nuts, chopped

1 cup of coconut oil

1 pastured egg

Filling:

2 cups broccoli florets, diced

5 pastured eggs

2/3 cup unsweetened coconut cream

1/4 teaspoon nutmeg

1 tsp. iodized sea salt

1 cup shredded goat's milk cheese

Directions:

1. Let your oven preheat at 400 degrees F. Grease an 8-inch pie pan with olive oil.
2. Combine all the ingredients for crust in a blender.
3. Add 1 teaspoon water if it is too dry.
4. Refrigerate this mixture for 1 hour to set after wrapping in a plastic sheet.
5. Spread the dough in the pie pan and press it firmly. Bake it for 10 mins.
6. Now decrease the oven's temperature to 350 degrees F.

7. Steam broccoli over boiling water for 3 minutes then drain it.
8. Whisk coconut cream with nutmeg, salt, and eggs in a bowl.
9. Add this mixture to the baked crust along with cheese and broccoli on top.
10. Return the pan to the oven for 40 minutes.
11. Slice and serve.

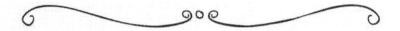

Brussels Sprouts, Kale, and Cabbage steaks
Prep + Cook time: 20 minutes | Serves: 2

Nutritional Info (per serving)

Calories	*Fat (g)*	*Protein (g)*	*Carbs (g)*
54	1.9	2.2	8.4

Ingredients

2 tbs. avocado oil

½ 1-inch-thick red cabbage slice

1/8 teaspoon plus 1 pinch sea salt, preferably iodized

1/4 red onion, thinly sliced

1/2 cup brussels sprouts, thinly sliced

3/4 cups chopped kale

1/2 tbs. freshly squeezed lemon juice

Extra-virgin olive oil (optional)

Directions:

1. Place a nonstick skillet over medium-high heat then add 1 tbsp oil.
2. Stir cabbage and sear the slices for 3 minutes per side.
3. Add pinch salt, mix well then transfer it to a plate.
4. Clean this pan and heat more avocado oil.
5. Stir in brussels sprouts and onion, sauté for 3 minutes.
6. Add lemon juice and kale. Stir cook for another 3 minutes.
7. Season with salt and serve warm.

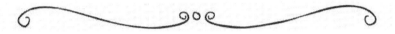

Brazilian Cheese Bread
Prep + Cook time: 30 minutes | Serves: 6-8

Nutritional Info (per serving)

Calories	*Fat (g)*	*Protein (g)*	*Carbs (g)*
175	17.9	1.7	4.9

Ingredients:

1 cup unsweetened coconut milk

½ cup avocado oil

1 tsp iodized sea salt

10 oz. (about 2 cups) cassava flour

2 pastured eggs

1 to 1½ cups grated Parmigiano-Reggiano cheese

Directions:

1. Let your oven preheat at 450 degrees F. Layer two baking sheet with wax paper.
2. Mix milk with oil and salt in a saucepan and cook it on a simmer.
3. Stir in flour when the milk starts to bubble, continue stirring the mixture meanwhile.
4. Beat this dough in an electric mixer for few minutes.
5. Whisk in eggs then cheese while beating on medium speed.
6. Scoop out the dough on the baking sheets to get 12 cookies per sheet.
7. Bake them for 15 minutes at 350 degrees F.
8. Rotate the baking sheet and bake again for 15 minutes until golden.

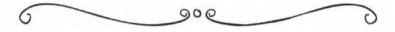

Carrot Cake Muffins

Prep + Cook time: 25 minutes | Serves: 2-4

Nutritional Info (per serving)

Calories	Fat (g)	Protein (g)	Carbs (g)
390	31.2	11.2	17.7

Ingredients:

1 1/4 cups blanched almond flour

2 tbs. coconut flour

1/2 teaspoon baking soda

1/8 teaspoon salt

1 1/2 teaspoons ground cinnamon

1/2 teaspoon ground ginger

1/4 teaspoon ground nutmeg

Two omega-3 or pastor and eggs or Vegan Eggs

1/3 cup MCT oil

2/3 cup coconut milk

1/3 cup Swerve

2 teaspoons vanilla

2 large carrots, grated

1/4 chopped walnuts

Directions:

1. Let your oven preheat at 350 degrees F. Layer muffin tray with paper liners.
2. Combined everything in a bowl using a mixing then fold in walnuts and carrots.
3. Divide the batter into muffin cups.
4. Bake them for 18 minutes until they are done.
5. Enjoy.

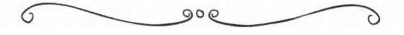

Coconut-Almond Flour Muffin
Prep + Cook time: 10 minutes | Serves: 1

Nutritional Info (per serving)

Calories	*Fat (g)*	*Protein (g)*	*Carbs (g)*
100	9.2	2.6	2.2

Ingredients:

1 tbs. coconut oil, melted

1 tbs. olive oil or macadamia nut oil

1 tbs. coconut flour

1 tbs. water

1 tbs. almond flour

1/2 teaspoon baking powder

1 pinch sea salt, preferably iodized

1 packet stevia

1 large pastured, beaten

Directions:

1. Combine everything together in a microwave mug until it forms a smooth batter
2. Place this mug in the microwave for 1 and a half minute at high temperature.
3. Serve.

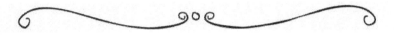

Orange Cranberry Muffins
Prep + Cook time: 25 minutes | Serves: 4-6

Nutritional Info (per serving)

Calories	*Fat (g)*	*Protein (g)*	*Carbs (g)*
239	18.2	7	11.6

Ingredients:

1/4 cup coconut flour

1/4 teaspoon sea salt, iodized

1/4 teaspoon baking soda

1/4 cup coconut oil, melted

1/4 cup xylitol

3 large pastured eggs

1 tbs. orange zest

1/2 cup dried, unsweetened cranberries

Directions:

1. Let your oven preheat at 350 degrees F.
2. Line a 6 cups muffin tray with paper liners.
3. Combine all the dry ingredients in a processor or a blender.
4. Then blend in eggs, zest and xylitol.
5. Fold in cranberries and divide the batter into the muffin cups.
6. Bake them for 20 mins until golden.
7. Serve.

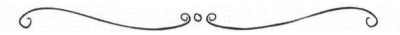

Flaxseed Muffin
Prep + Cook time: 10 minutes | Serves: 1

Nutritional Info (per serving)

Calories	Fat (g)	Protein (g)	Carbs (g)
326	22.9	13.3	11.8

Ingredients:

1/4 cup ground flaxseed

1 teaspoon cinnamon

1 large pastured egg

1 tbs. extra-virgin coconut oil, melted

1 teaspoon aluminum-free baking powder

1 packet stevia

Directions:

1. Combine everything together in a microwave mug until it forms a smooth batter
2. Place this mug in the microwave for 1 and a half minute at high temperature.
3. Serve.

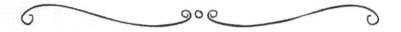

Green Egg Muffins

Prep + Cook time: 55 minutes | Serves: 4-6

Nutritional Info (per serving)

Calories	*Fat (g)*	*Protein (g)*	*Carbs (g)*
398	26.9	29.1	9.3

Ingredients:

1-pound Diestel Farms Turkey Sausage

10-ounce chopped organic frozen spinach

5 pastured eggs

2 tbs. olive oil or perilla oil

2 cloves garlic, peeled

2 tbs. Italian seasoning

2 tbs. dried minced onion

1/2 teaspoon sea salt, preferably iodized

1/2 teaspoon cracked black pepper

Directions:

1. Let your oven preheat at 350 degrees F. layer a muffin tray with paper liner.
2. Add crumbled sausage to a skillet and sauté it for 10 minutes then set it aside.

3. Defrost the spinach in the microwave in a covered bowl.
4. Drain the spinach and squeeze out all the water from it.
5. Blend the spinach with eggs, garlic, oil, onion, salt, Italian seasoning and black pepper in a blender.
6. Fold in the sautéed sausage this divide the batter into the muffin cups.
7. Bake them for 35 minutes.
8. Serve.

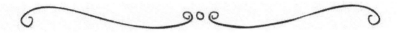

Plantain Pancakes
Prep + Cook time: 15 minutes | Serves: 4

Nutritional Info (per serving)

Calories	*Fat (g)*	*Protein (g)*	*Carbs (g)*
322	21.3	7.2	44.8

Ingredients:

2 large green plantains, peeled and diced

2 teaspoons vanilla essence

5 tbs. coconut oil

4 large pastured eggs

1/4 cuperythritol

1/8 teaspoon sea salt, iodized

1/2 teaspoon baking soda

Directions:

1. Puree the plantain in a blender then whisk in eggs.
2. Beat in vanilla essence, erythritol, salt, baking soda, and 3 tbsp coconut oil.

3. Blend the mixture for about 3 minutes until smooth.
4. Place a greased griddle pan over medium heat.
5. Pour ½ cup batter into the hot pan and cook for 2 minutes per side.
6. Make more cakes using this batter.
7. Enjoy.

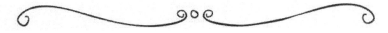

Cassava Flour Waffles
Prep + Cook time: 15 minutes | Serves: 4

Nutritional Info (per serving)

Calories	*Fat (g)*	*Protein (g)*	*Carbs (g)*
104	4.2	6.6	11

Ingredients:

4 pastured eggs

1/4 cup Vital Proteins marine collagen

1/2 cup cassava flour

1/2 cup extra-virgin coconut oil, melted

1 tbs. Manuka honey

1/2 teaspoon baking soda

1/4 teaspoon salt

One 12oz. package Trader Joe's frozen wild blueberries

Directions:

1. Preheat waffle iron on medium heat.
2. Whisk eggs with all the ingredients using a mixer to get a smooth batter.

3. Ladle ¼ cup batter into the waffle iron and cook it as per machine's instructions.
4. Make more waffles in this way.
5. Top each waffle with ¼ cup blueberries.
6. Enjoy.

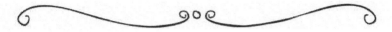

Spinach Pancakes with Blueberries
Prep + Cook time: 15 minutes | Serves: 4-6

Nutritional Info (per serving)

Calories	*Fat (g)*	*Protein (g)*	*Carbs (g)*
308	16.2	9	32.6

Ingredients:

10oz clean, fresh spinach

2 pastured raised eggs

1 cup full fat coconut milk

3/4 cup hemp milk, unsweetened

9 tbsp almond flour

9 tbsp cassava flour

2 scoops marine collagen

1 nutmeg, grated

1/2 tsp sea salt

frozen wild blueberries for serving

pepper

Directions:

1. Puree the spinach in a blender and blend with eggs, nutmeg, salt, and pepper.

2. Pour this mixture into a bowl and stir flour and marine collagen.
3. Place a greased griddle pan over medium heat.
4. Pour ¼ cup of more batter into the pan and cook it for 2 minutes per side.
5. Make as many as seven pancakes out of this batter.
6. Stir cook blueberries in pan for 3 minutes.
7. Pour these berries over the pancakes.
8. Enjoy.

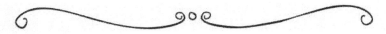

Sun Kissed Bread
Prep + Cook time: 35 minutes | Serves: 2-4

Nutritional Info (per serving)

Calories	Fat (g)	Protein (g)	Carbs (g)
524	33.8	2.1	54.6

Ingredients:

425g cassava flour

425g sweet potato puree

2/3 cups extra virgin olive oil

2/3 cup water, room temperature

1 tsp sea salt

2 tsp Turmeric Tonic

1/2 tsp turmeric powder

Directions:

1. Let your oven preheat at 400 degrees F.

2. Combine all the ingredients in a processor or blender to get a smooth dough.
3. Make small 2 inches balls out of this dough.
4. Place them in a baking sheet and bake them for 30 minutes.
5. Enjoy.

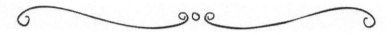

Cinnamon Muffins

Prep + Cook time: 25 minutes | Serves: 2-4

Nutritional Info (per serving)

Calories	Fat (g)	Protein (g)	Carbs (g)
135	4.6	15.1	11.6

Ingredients:

2 cups, 2 Tbsp oat flour

1 Tbsp baking powder

1/2 tsp salt

2 tsp cinnamon

1/4 tsp vanilla bean powder

11oz silken tofu, diced

1/2 cup melted vegan butter

1/2 tsp apple cider vinegar

1 shot freshly brewed espresso

1 cup of coconut sugar

topping: 1 Tbsp cinnamon sugar mix

2 tsp vegan butter: for greasing a muffin tin

Directions:

1. Let your oven preheat at 400 degrees F.
2. Grease a muffin tray with 2 tsp butter.

3. Grind rolled oats with flour in a blender then add baking powder, cinnamon, and salt. Transfer the mixture to a bowl.
4. Beat tofu, vinegar, melted butter, sugar and espresso in a blender.
5. Mix both the wet and dry mixtures until smooth.
6. Divide the batter into the muffin cups.
7. Bake them for 12 minutes then at 350 degrees for 8 minutes.
8. Serve.

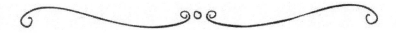

Pear & Oat Scones

Prep + Cook time: 30 minutes | Serves: 10-12

Nutritional Info (per serving)

Calories	*Fat (g)*	*Protein (g)*	*Carbs (g)*
396	24.1	7.7	39

Ingredients:

1 cup oat flour

1 cup old-fashioned oats

⅓cup of coconut sugar

2-1/4 tsp baking powder

1 tsp ground cardamom

¼ tsp fine sea salt

⅓ cup solid coconut oil, cut into chunks

1 large egg

2 tbsp almond milk

1-1/4 cups chopped fresh pears

Directions:

1. Let your oven preheat at 400 degrees F. Layer a baking sheet with wax paper.
2. Combine oat flour with sugar, oats, salt, baking powder and cardamom in a bowl.
3. Cut in coconut oil and blend the mixture get a crumbly mixture.
4. Whisk in milk and egg. Mix well then fold in pears.
5. Roll the dough in a floured surface and cut twelve ½ inch thick wedges out of it.
6. Arrange the wedges in the baking sheet and bake them for 22 minutes.
7. Serve.

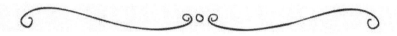

Baked Strawberry Pie
Prep + Cook time: 35 minutes | Serves: 2-3

Nutritional Info (per serving)

Calories	Fat (g)	Protein (g)	Carbs (g)
298	21	7.2	20.7

Ingredients:

1/8 cup cassava flour	1/8 cup almond flour
1/2 teaspoon vanilla	1/8 teaspoon baking soda
1 cup strawberries, slices	2 drops stevia, liquid
1 pastured egg	1/2 teaspoon salt
1/2 tbs. coconut oil, melted	3 ½ ounces almond milk
1/8 cup coconut flour	1/4 teaspoon baking powder

1 teaspoon Swerve powder,
to drizzle

Directions:

1. Let your oven preheat 350 degrees F. Layer a 6-inch pie dish with coconut oil.
2. Beat all the wet ingredients then stir in remaining dry ingredients.
3. Mix well until smooth then transfer the batter into the pie dish.
4. Top it with half of the strawberry slices and drizzle swerve on top.
5. Bake, the pie for 20-25 until it is cooked inside out, bake more if needed.
6. Allow it to cool then garnish with remaining strawberry slices.
7. Serve.

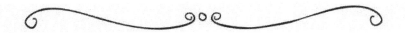

Buckwheat Porridge
Prep + Cook time: 25 minutes | Serves: 2-4

Nutritional Info (per serving)

Calories	Fat (g)	Protein (g)	Carbs (g)
477	32	8.1	48.6

Ingredients:

1 cup of buckwheat groats

2 cups of almond milk

1 cup of water

2 ripe bananas

1 tbs. manuka honey

2 teaspoons of cinnamon

| 1 tbs. of almond butter | 1 tbs. of baobab powder |

Directions:

1. Cook the buckwheat in 1 cup boiling water until it is al dente.
2. Add the bananas, honey, and cinnamon.
3. Once the water is dried up, then add the almond milk.
4. Stir cook the mixture for 20 minutes in a simmer.
5. Add the almond butter and baobab powder.
6. Serve.

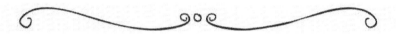

Crusty Egg Quiche
Prep + Cook time: 45 minutes | Serves: 2-4

Nutritional Info (per serving)

Calories	*Fat (g)*	*Protein (g)*	*Carbs (g)*
502	35.7	23.9	22.2

Ingredients:

Quiche Crust

2 cups almond flour	¾ tsp baking soda
½ tsp salt	¾ cup melted coconut oil
1.5 Tbsp water	

Quiche Filling

| ½ red onion, finely diced | 2 handfuls of baby spinach, chopped |
| 2 garlic cloves | |

½ cup red olives, pitted and sliced

4 organic eggs

¼ cup nutritional yeast

2 Tbsp vegetable broth

Pepper to taste

Directions:

1. Let your oven preheat at 350 degrees F. layer the muffin tray with the muffin liners.
2. Combine all the crust ingredients in a mixer to get a crumbly mixture.
3. Divide the mixture into the muffin liners and press it against their bottom.
4. Poke 2 to 3 holes in the bottom using a fork and bake them for 15 minutes.
5. Meanwhile, sauté onion in a greased pan for 5 minutes then add garlic.
6. Stir cook for 2 minutes then add spinach. Cook for 5 minutes.
7. Turn of its heat then adds olives.
8. Whisk eggs with yeast, broth, and pepper in a bowl until foamy.
9. Pour the mixture into the baked crusts then top them with vegetable mixture.
10. Bake again for 20 minutes.
11. Enjoy.

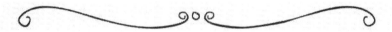

Dijon Spinach Strata

Prep + Cook time: 35 minutes | Serves: 4

Nutritional Info (per serving)

Calories	*Fat (g)*	*Protein (g)*	*Carbs (g)*

Ingredients:

1 tsp olive oil	3/4 tsp salt
1 tsp Dijon mustard	1/4 tsp black pepper
1 garlic clove, chopped or minced	4 cups baby spinach
	4 oz. feta cheese, crumbled
8 large eggs	

Directions:

1. Let your oven preheat at 350 degrees F.
2. Whisk eggs and olive oil with pepper in a medium bowl.
3. Grease a pie dish with cooking oil and spread spinach leaves in it.
4. Top it with egg mixture and bake it with for 35 minutes in the preheated oven.
5. Garnish with bacon.
6. Serve.

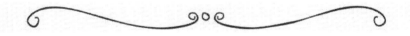

Coconut Waffles
Prep + Cook time: 15 minutes | Serves: 2-4

Nutritional Info (per serving)

Calories	*Fat (g)*	*Protein (g)*	*Carbs (g)*
168	11.3	3.2	14.3

Ingredients:

2 tbsp ground chia or flax seeds

1 large banana, mashed well

1 1/4 cups non-dairy milk

1/4 cup melted coconut oil

2 tbsp maple syrup + more for serving

1 tsp vanilla extract

1 cup almond meal

1 cup gluten-free oat flour

1/4 cup sweet sorghum flour

1 tbsp baking powder

1/2 tbsp arrowroot powder

1 tsp ground cinnamon

1/2 cup shredded, unsweetened coconut

pinch of salt

Directions:

1. Preheat your waffle iron on medium heat.
2. Combine chia ground, maple syrup, vanilla extract, banana mash and milk in any container.
3. Combine rest of the ingredients in a separate bowl.
4. Stir in the banana mixture and mix them well until smooth.
5. Layer the inside of the waffle iron with oil and pour 1/2 cup batter into it.
6. Cook the waffle as per the machine's instructions for 4 minutes.
7. Make more waffles using the same steps.
8. Garnish with coconut shred and maple syrup.

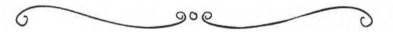

Vegan Pumpkin Waffles
Prep + Cook time: 15 minutes | Serves: 2-4

Nutritional Info (per serving)

Calories	Fat (g)	Protein (g)	Carbs (g)
376	12.1	13	57.7

Ingredients:

Dry ingredients:

1 1/2 cups rolled oats

1 tsp baking powder

1/4 tsp salt

1/4 tsp pumpkin pie spice

1/4 cup raw pumpkin seeds

Wet Ingredients:

1 Tbsp vegan butter, melted (optional)

1/2 cup pumpkin puree, unsweetened

1/2 tsp fresh orange zest

1/4 cup non-dairy milk

1 Tbsp maple syrup, grade B

Directions:

1. Let the waffle iron preheat at medium heat.
2. Grind oats with pumpkin seeds in a processor and blend it with other dry ingredients.
3. Transfer this mixture to a bowl then blend the remaining ingredients.
4. Pour the wet mixture into the pumpkin seeds mixture and mix well.
5. Grease the waffle iron with some coconut oil and pour ¼ cup of the batter in it.
6. Cook them waffle as per machine's instructions.

7. Use more batter to make more waffles.
8. Enjoy.

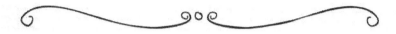

Pecan Walnut Cereal

Prep + Cook time: 15 minutes | Serves: 1

Nutritional Info (per serving)

Calories	*Fat (g)*	*Protein (g)*	*Carbs (g)*
108	6.4	4.9	8.1

Ingredients:

¼ cup finely chopped walnuts and pecans

¼ cup unsweetened coconut flakes

2 tbs. flax seed meal

2 tbs. coconut flour

1 tbs. chia seeds

½ teaspoon cinnamon

½ teaspoon vanilla bean powder

⅛ teaspoon kosher salt

1 cup non-dairy milk of choice

1-2 tbs. date paste

Directions:

1. Take a saucepan and warm up the milk in it.
2. Toss in all the ingredients and cook until it thickens.
3. Garnish as desired.
4. Enjoy.

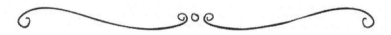

Avocado Smoothie Bowl

Prep + Cook time: 15 minutes | Serves: 1

Nutritional Info (per serving)

Calories	*Fat (g)*	*Protein (g)*	*Carbs (g)*
291	19.1	8.9	38.5

Ingredients:

3 oz. ripe avocado flesh

3 oz. full-fat coconut milk

3 oz. water

3 oz. of ice

1 1/2 tbsp flax meal

1 tbsp erythritol

1 tsp Matcha (optional)

1/4 tsp vanilla extract

1/4 tsp liquid stevia

medium pinch of salt

1 tbsp extra virgin olive oil

Directions:

1. Blend everything for the smoothie in a blender.
2. Transfer the smoothie to a serving bowl.
3. Top it with blueberries, coconut flakes, and pistachios.
4. Enjoy.

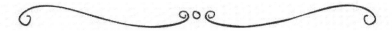

Smoothie Recipes

Purple Smoothie

Prep + Cook time: 5 minutes | Serves: 1

Nutritional Info (per serving)

Calories	*Fat (g)*	*Protein (g)*	*Carbs (g)*
386	22.6	5.6	45.8

Ingredients:

¾ cup coconut or almond milk

¼ cup of coconut yogurt (unsweetened)

1 large handful of baby spinach

¼ cup purple sweet potato (boiled and cooled, skin removed)

1 cup of frozen berries

1-2 drops liquid stevia if desired

Directions:

1. Put everything into a clean blender jar.
2. Pulse the blender for 30 seconds to blend everything together.
3. Enjoy.

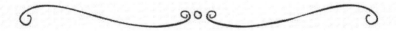

Hemp Seed Protein Smoothie

Prep + Cook time: 5 minutes | Serves: 1

Nutritional Info (per serving)

Calories	Fat (g)	Protein (g)	Carbs (g)
287	6.2	25.7	37.2

Ingredients:

2 cups of filtered tap water

2 cups organic baby spinach leaves

1 cup organic baby kale leaves

2 tbs. Nutiva Hemp Protein

2 Droppers of Sweet Leaf Sweet Drops Sweetener, liquid stevia

1 cup of ice

Directions:

4. Put everything into a clean blender jar.
5. Pulse the blender for 30 seconds to blend everything together.
6. Enjoy.

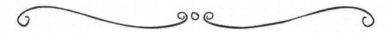

Berry-Licious Smoothie
Prep + Cook time: 5 minutes | Serves: 1

Nutritional Info (per serving)

Calories	Fat (g)	Protein (g)	Carbs (g)
226	0.7	2.1	57.3

Ingredients:

1 cup frozen raspberries   1 cup frozen blueberries

1 ripe banana

1 1/2 cups coconut milk

1 thumb fresh turmeric

1 thumb fresh ginger

Directions:

1. Put everything into a clean blender jar.
2. Pulse the blender for 30 seconds to blend everything together.
3. Enjoy.

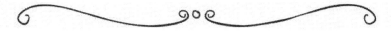

Triple Berry Smoothie

Prep + Cook time: 5 minutes | Serves: 1

Nutritional Info (per serving)

Calories	Fat (g)	Protein (g)	Carbs (g)
640	5.2	6.4	155.3

Ingredients:

2 medium bananas, sliced and frozen

1 cup unsweetened almond milk

1 cup of frozen strawberries

1 cup frozen blueberries

1 cup frozen raspberries

Directions:

1. Put everything into a clean blender jar.
2. Pulse the blender for 30 seconds to blend everything together.

3. Enjoy.

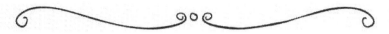

Banana Chia Smoothie
Prep + Cook time: 5 minutes | Serves: 2

Nutritional Info (per serving)

Calories	*Fat (g)*	*Protein (g)*	*Carbs (g)*
388	12.3	8.2	69.6

Ingredients:

2 tbs. chia seeds

1 ½ cups unsweetened almond milk, divided

3 medium bananas, sliced and frozen

1 ½ cups frozen blueberries

Directions:

1. Soak chia seeds in almond milk for 15- 30 minutes.
2. Put everything into a clean blender jar.
3. Pulse the blender for 30 seconds to blend everything together.
4. Enjoy.

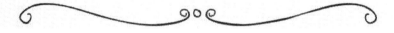

Red, White & Blue Smoothie
Prep + Cook time: 5 minutes | Serves: 2

Nutritional Info (per serving)

Calories	Fat (g)	Protein (g)	Carbs (g)
504	25.9	8.3	67.3

Ingredients:

Red Smoothie:

1 cup frozen raspberries

1 cup of frozen strawberries

1 cup pomegranate juice (or coconut water)

juice from half a lemon

White Smoothie:

1/2 cup frozen pineapple

1/2 cup shredded coconut

2 frozen bananas (sliced)

1 can of coconut milk

2 tbs. of hemp seeds

Blue Smoothie:

1 cup frozen blueberries

2 dates (pitted)

2 tbs. chia seeds

1 cup of pomegranate juice (or coconut water)

Directions:

1. First put everything for the red smoothie into a clean blender jar.
2. Pulse the blender for 30 seconds to blend everything together.
3. Fill 1/3 of the serving glass/es with this smoothie.
4. Put everything for white smoothie in to the blender jar.

5. Pulse the blender for 30 seconds to blend everything together.
6. Fill 1/3 of the serving glass/es with this smoothie.
7. Put everything for blue smoothie in to the blender jar.
8. Pulse the blender for 30 seconds to blend everything together.
9. Fill 1/3 of the serving glass/es with this smoothie.
10. Enjoy.

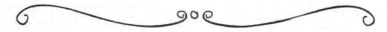

Strawberry Butter Smoothie
Prep + Cook time: 5 minutes | Serves: 1

Nutritional Info (per serving)

Calories	*Fat (g)*	*Protein (g)*	*Carbs (g)*
505	6.7	5.6	116.6

Ingredients:

3 medium bananas, sliced and frozen

1 cup unsweetened almond milk

2 cups frozen strawberries

¼ cup unsalted, natural coconut butter

Directions:

1. Put everything into a clean blender jar.
2. Pulse the blender for 30 seconds to blend everything together.
3. Enjoy.

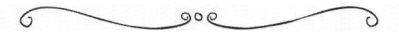

Strawberry Coconut Milkshake

Prep + Cook time: 5 minutes | Serves: 1

Nutritional Info (per serving)

Calories	*Fat (g)*	*Protein (g)*	*Carbs (g)*
364	0.9	2.6	93.8

Ingredients:

2 medium bananas, sliced and frozen

1 can coconut milk (13.66 oz.)

1cup of frozen strawberries

2-3 tbs. pure maple syrup

Directions:

1. Put everything into a clean blender jar.
2. Pulse the blender for 30 seconds to blend everything together.
3. Enjoy.

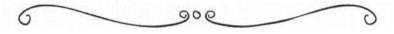

Mocha Frappe

Prep + Cook time: 5 minutes | Serves: 1

Nutritional Info (per serving)

Calories	*Fat (g)*	*Protein (g)*	*Carbs (g)*
454	4.1	6.8	111.7

Ingredients:

Mocha Frappe

½ cup cold coffee

4 medium bananas, sliced and frozen

½ cup unsweetened almond milk

1 tbs. unsweetened cocoa powder

Optional Toppings

Coconut whip, chocolate syrup, and chocolate curls

Directions:

1. Put everything into a clean blender jar.
2. Pulse the blender for 30 seconds to blend everything together.
3. Enjoy.

Coffee Coconut Frappuccino
Prep + Cook time: 5 minutes | Serves: 1

Nutritional Info (per serving)

Calories	*Fat (g)*	*Protein (g)*	*Carbs (g)*
487	29.4	5.5	60.6

Ingredients:

Frappuccino

1 can light coconut milk (13-14 oz.)

½ cup cold coffee

2 medium bananas, sliced and frozen

Optional toppings

Toasted coconut, coconut whip

Directions:

1. Put everything into a clean blender jar.
2. Pulse the blender for 30 seconds to blend everything together.
3. Top the smoothie with coconut whip cream, and toasted coconut.
4. Enjoy.

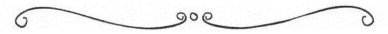

Mango Chia Seed Smoothie
Prep + Cook time: 5 minutes | Serves: 1

Nutritional Info (per serving)

Calories	*Fat (g)*	*Protein (g)*	*Carbs (g)*
537	11.6	9.1	112.3

Ingredients:

2 tbs. chia seeds

1 ½ cups unsweetened almond milk, divided

2 medium bananas, sliced and frozen

2 cups frozen mango chunks

Directions:

1. Soak the chia seeds in milk for 15-30 minutes.
2. Put everything into a clean blender jar.

3. Pulse the blender for 30 seconds to blend everything together.
4. Enjoy.

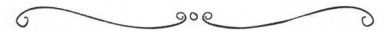

Frozen fruit smoothie
Prep + Cook time: 5 minutes | Serves: 1

Nutritional Info (per serving)

Calories	Fat (g)	Protein (g)	Carbs (g)
275	1.8	6.7	59.8

Ingredients:

1–2 cup chopped deseeded watermelon

1 cup of frozen mixed berries

1 banana

1/4 c coconut milk/cream or yogurt

8 oz. sparkling lime water

Directions:

1. Put everything into a clean blender jar.
2. Pulse the blender for 30 seconds to blend everything together.
3. Enjoy.

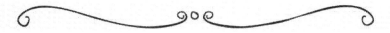

Peppermint Mocha Frappuccino
Prep + Cook time: 5 minutes | Serves: 1

Nutritional Info (per serving)

Calories	Fat (g)	Protein (g)	Carbs (g)

454	4.1	6.8	111.7

Ingredients:

Frappuccino

½ cup cold coffee

4 medium bananas, sliced and frozen

½ cup unsweetened almond milk

1 tbs. unsweetened cocoa powder

¼ teaspoon pure peppermint extract

Optional Toppings

Dairy-free whipped topping, chocolate, or your favorite toppings

Directions:

1. Put everything into a clean blender jar.
2. Pulse the blender for 30 seconds to blend everything together.
3. Garnish the smoothie with desired toppings.
4. Enjoy.

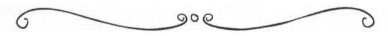

Strawberry Almond Butter Smoothie
Prep + Cook time: 5 minutes | Serves: 2

Nutritional Info (per serving)

Calories	*Fat (g)*	*Protein (g)*	*Carbs (g)*
407	18.3	7.4	61.4

Ingredients:

3 medium bananas, sliced and frozen

1 cup unsweetened almond milk

2 cups frozen strawberries

¼ cup unsalted, natural almond butter

Directions:

1. Put everything into a clean blender jar.
2. Pulse the blender for 30 seconds to blend everything together.
3. Enjoy.

Sweet Potato Ginger Smoothie
Prep + Cook time: 5 minutes | Serves: 1

Nutritional Info (per serving)

Calories	*Fat (g)*	*Protein (g)*	*Carbs (g)*
252	14.8	3.9	28.5

Ingredients:

½ cup cooked the sweet potato, cold

¼ cup full-fat canned coconut milk

2 tbsp water

3 tsp fresh ginger - grated

¼ tsp ground cinnamon

¼ tsp vanilla essence

¼ tsp lemon juice

Directions:

1. Put everything into a clean blender jar.
2. Pulse the blender for 30 seconds to blend everything together.
3. Enjoy.

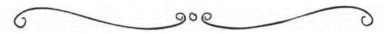

Chocolate Avocado Green Smoothie

Prep + Cook time: 5 minutes | Serves: 2

Nutritional Info (per serving)

Calories	Fat (g)	Protein (g)	Carbs (g)
462	44.5	7.5	19

Ingredients:

1/2 a ripe avocado, cored and peeled

5 or 6 baby carrots, peeled, diced

1 cup of spinach, washed

3 tbs. unsweetened cocoa powder

1 tbs. almond butter

1/2 teaspoon vanilla extract

A pinch of cayenne

1 cup of chocolate almond milk

2-4 ice cubes, as needed

Optional 1 teaspoon honey, or to taste

Directions:

1. Put everything into a clean blender jar.

2. Pulse the blender for 30 seconds or more to blend everything together.
3. Enjoy.

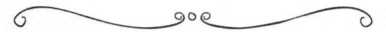

Chicory Breve Latte

Prep + Cook time: 5 minutes | Serves: 4

Nutritional Info (per serving)

Calories	*Fat (g)*	*Protein (g)*	*Carbs (g)*
472	25.9	8	52.8

Ingredients:

8 ounces hot chicory coffee

4 ounces unsweetened coconut milk

4 ounces unsweetened coconut cream

2 teaspoons raw honey

Directions:

1. Put everything into a clean blender jar.
2. Pulse the blender for 30 seconds to blend everything together.
3. Enjoy.

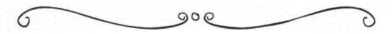

Green Detox Smoothie

Prep + Cook time: 5 minutes | Serves: 1

Nutritional Info (per serving)

Calories	*Fat (g)*	*Protein (g)*	*Carbs (g)*

246	11.8	5.4	34.8

Ingredients:

1/4 - 1/2 cup almond milk

2 cups fresh baby spinach leaves, lightly packed

1 cup frozen pineapple, chopped

1 medium carrot, peeled then chopped

1 clementine or 1/2 orange, juice only

1 teaspoon chia seeds

1/2 teaspoon minced ginger

6 ice cubes

Directions:

1. Put everything into a clean blender jar.
2. Pulse the blender for 30 seconds to blend everything together.
3. Enjoy.

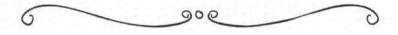

Green Breakfast Smoothie
Prep + Cook time: 5 minutes | Serves: 1

Nutritional Info (per serving)

Calories	Fat (g)	Protein (g)	Carbs (g)
216	19.8	2.6	10.8

Ingredients:

1 cup of chopped romaine lettuce

1/2 cup of baby spinach

1 mint spring with stem

1/2 avocado, flesh only

4 tbs. lemon juice

3 to 6 drops of stevia extract

4 cup of ice cubes

1 cup of water

Directions:

1. Put everything into a clean blender jar.
2. Pulse the blender for 30 seconds to blend everything together.
3. Enjoy.

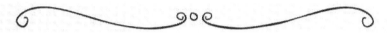

Tropical Turmeric Smoothie

Prep + Cook time: 5 minutes | Serves: 1

Nutritional Info (per serving)

Calories	*Fat (g)*	*Protein (g)*	*Carbs (g)*
375	1.2	4.8	94.8

Ingredients:

1 orange, peeled (juice)

1 peeled and sliced frozen banana

1/2 cup frozen pineapple chunks

1/2 cup frozen mango chunks

1/2 teaspoon ground turmeric

1 carrot, grated

1/2 cup ice cubes

Directions:

1. Put everything into a clean blender jar.

2. Pulse the blender for 30 seconds to blend everything together.
3. Enjoy.

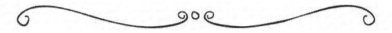

Dragon Fruit Smoothie
Prep + Cook time: 5 minutes | Serves: 1

Nutritional Info (per serving)

Calories	*Fat (g)*	*Protein (g)*	*Carbs (g)*
301	11.2	11.1	42.4

Ingredients:

1 orange, peeled

1 cup frozen peach chunks

1 frozen dragon fruit
(pitaya) pack

1 tbs. hemp hearts

1/3 cup coconut yogurt

Directions:

1. Put everything into a clean blender jar.
2. Pulse the blender for 30 seconds to blend everything together.
3. Enjoy.

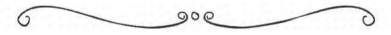

Banana Ginger Green Smoothie
Prep + Cook time: 5 minutes | Serves: 1

Nutritional Info (per serving)

Calories	Fat (g)	Protein (g)	Carbs (g)
215	0.5	5.6	54.4

Ingredients:

1 cup of water

1 ripe banana (with black speckles)

2 large handfuls baby spinach

1-inch fresh ginger root

4 large Medjool dates, pitted

12 ice cubes

Directions:

1. Put everything into a clean blender jar.
2. Pulse the blender for 30 seconds to blend everything together.
3. Enjoy.

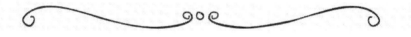

Oatmeal Breakfast Smoothie

Prep + Cook time: 5 minutes | Serves: 4

Nutritional Info (per serving)

Calories	Fat (g)	Protein (g)	Carbs (g)
183	2.1	6	37.8

Ingredients

3/4 cup rolled oats, gluten free , soaked

2 cups freshly cubed pineapple

2 cups mixed frozen berries

6" piece of cucumber

6 leaves Swiss Chard

5 cups filtered water

Stevia to taste

Directions:

1. Put everything into a clean blender jar.
2. Pulse the blender for 30 seconds to blend everything together.
3. Enjoy.

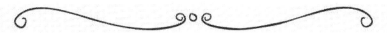

Berry Oatmeal Breakfast Smoothie
Prep + Cook time: 5 minutes | Serves: 1

Nutritional Info (per serving)

Calories	*Fat (g)*	*Protein (g)*	*Carbs (g)*
217	2.8	4.7	40.7

Ingredients:

1 cup of frozen berries (raspberries, strawberries, blueberries)

1 Tangelo or Orange, peeled and deseeded

1/3 cup gluten free oatmeal

4 ice cubes

1 cup of water

Directions:

1. Put everything into a clean blender jar.

2. Pulse the blender for 30 seconds to blend everything together.
3. Enjoy.

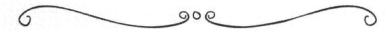

Chocolate Cherry Smoothie
Prep + Cook time: 5 minutes | Serves: 1

Nutritional Info (per serving)

Calories	Fat (g)	Protein (g)	Carbs (g)
246	8.2	2.6	40.6

Ingredients:

2 cups unsweetened almond milk

2 cups frozen dark sweet cherries

1 ripe banana

2 tbs. raw cacao nibs

2 ice cubes

1/2 teaspoon vanilla extract

Directions:

1. Put everything into a clean blender jar.
2. Pulse the blender for 30 seconds to blend everything together.
3. Enjoy.

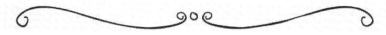

Chocolate Coconut Smoothie
Prep + Cook time: 5 minutes | Serves: 1

Nutritional Info (per serving)

Calories	Fat (g)	Protein (g)	Carbs (g)
497	30.1	17.5	43

Ingredients:

1 cup of coconut meat

1 cup of coconut water

1 tbs. raw cacao powder

1/2 teaspoon ground cinnamon

1/4 teaspoon vanilla stevia

4 ice cubes

Directions:

1. Put everything into a clean blender jar.
2. Pulse the blender for 30 seconds to blend everything together.
3. Enjoy.

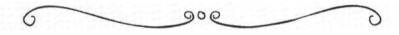

Green Lemonade

Prep + Cook time: 5 minutes | Serves: 1

Nutritional Info (per serving)

Calories	Fat (g)	Protein (g)	Carbs (g)
385	1.5	3.6	101.7

Ingredients:

1 1/2-inch piece ginger root

1 large 12" English cucumber, peeled and diced

3 Granny Smith apples, cored, peeled and diced

1 lemon, zest

Directions:

1. Put everything into a clean blender jar.
2. Pulse the blender for 30 seconds to blend everything together.
3. Enjoy.

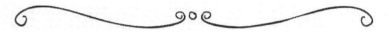

Flu Elixir

Prep + Cook time: 5 minutes | Serves: 1

Nutritional Info (per serving)

Calories	Fat (g)	Protein (g)	Carbs (g)
223	1	5.5	56.4

Ingredients:

1 cup green cabbage, chopped

1 cup English cucumber, chopped

1 cup packed baby spinach

1 cup fresh pineapple, cubed

2 cups seedless watermelon, cubed

1-inch ginger root

1-inch turmeric root

1/2 lemon, 2/3 of skin removed

Directions:

1. Put everything into a clean blender jar.
2. Pulse the blender for 30 seconds to blend everything together.
3. Enjoy.

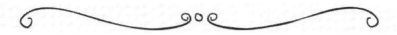

Dandelion Green Juice

Prep + Cook time: 5 minutes | Serves: 1

Nutritional Info (per serving)

Calories	Fat (g)	Protein (g)	Carbs (g)
183	0.9	2.6	46.9

Ingredients:

1 large bundle of dandelion

1-inch of ginger root

1 whole lemon unpeeled

1/2 of a large pineapple, peeled

1 granny smith apple, cored and peeled

Directions:

1. Put everything into a clean blender jar.
2. Pulse the blender for 30 seconds to blend everything together.
3. Enjoy.

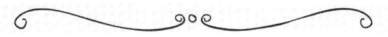

Blueberry Pear Smoothie

Prep + Cook time: 5 minutes | Serves: 1

Nutritional Info (per serving)

Calories	Fat (g)	Protein (g)	Carbs (g)
441	8.2	8.6	93.5

Ingredients:

2 cups frozen blueberries

1 Asian pear, chopped & deseeded

3 pitted dates

2 tbs. Hemp seeds

2 cups of water

Directions:

1. Put everything into a clean blender jar.
2. Pulse the blender for 30 seconds to blend everything together.
3. Enjoy.

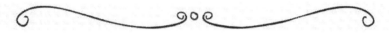

Poultry Recipes

Chicken Broccoli

Prep + Cook time: 25 minutes | Serves: 2

Nutritional Info (per serving)

Calories	*Fat (g)*	*Protein (g)*	*Carbs (g)*
355	11.5	39.9	16.2

Ingredients:

3/4-pound pastured chicken breast, cubed

3 scallion whites, thinly sliced

2 cloves garlic, minced and divided

1 inch peeled fresh ginger, minced and divided

2 tbs. coconut aminos

1 tbs. golden monk fruit sweetener

1 tbs. arrowroot starch

Sea salt and black pepper

1 tbs. dry sherry or cooking wine

1 tbs. sesame oil

3 tbs. avocado oil

2 broccoli crowns, cut into florets

2 broccoli stalks, trimmed and sliced

Directions:

1. Mix the chicken with half of the ginger, and garlic, scallions, sweetener, coconut aminos, arrowroot starch, dry sherry, salt and 1 tbs. sesame oil in a bowl.
2. Cover the chicken and marinate it for 15 minutes at room temperature.
3. Preheat 1 tbs. avocado oil in a large skillet on medium heat.

4. Toss in broccoli stems and sauté for 30 seconds.
5. Stir in the florets, 2 tbs. water, salt, pepper, and remaining ginger and garlic.
6. Stir cook for 2 minutes then transfers the mixture to a plate.
7. Add the remaining avocado oil to the same pan and heat it.
8. Stir in chicken along with its marinade
9. Sauté the chicken for 3 minutes until its golden brown.
10. Toss the broccoli back into the pan along with ¼ cup water.
11. Serve warm.

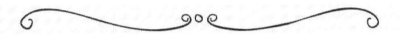

Chicken Mushroom Soup
Prep + Cook time: 45 minutes | Serves: 4

Nutritional Info (per serving)

Calories	Fat (g)	Protein (g)	Carbs (g)
418	24.8	42.5	7.1

Ingredients:

4 chicken thighs or drumsticks with bones (pasture raised chicken)

1 can full-fat coconut milk

1 stick lemongrass, smashed and cut in 1-2-inch pieces

1 thumb size or a bigger piece of ginger, cut in smaller pieces

1 tbs. coriander seeds

2 big garlic cloves

1 tbs. fish sauce

1 oz. dry shiitake mushrooms

1 bunch fresh cilantro

salt and pepper to taste

1 organic lime

avocado oil

Directions:

1. Mash the ginger, garlic, coriander seeds and lemon grass in a mortar using a pestle.
2. Stir fry this mixture for 30 seconds in a pot with heated avocado oil
3. Add chicken with salt and spices. Cook it until golden brown.
4. Pour in coconut milk, fish sauce and enough water to cover the chicken.
5. Cook the soup for 30 minutes on low simmer.
6. Adjust seasoning with salt and lime.
7. Strain the cooked soup and discard the ginger and lemongrass.
8. Remove chicken meat from the bones then return the chicken and mushrooms to the soup.
9. Garnish with cilantro.
10. Serve warm.

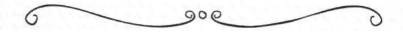

Italian Balsamic Chicken Salad
Prep + Cook time: 40 minutes | Serves: 2

Nutritional Info (per serving)

Calories	*Fat (g)*	*Protein (g)*	*Carbs (g)*
355	32.6	14.9	2.5

Ingredients:

1 romaine lettuce, rinsed

1 Boston lettuce, rinsed

2 pasture raised chicken breasts

1 handful of pitted, black olives

1 tbs. balsamic vinaigrette

1 teaspoon Dijon mustard

about 4 medium button or cremini mushrooms, sliced with a mandolin

4 tbs. extra virgin olive oil

salt and pepper to taste

1 teaspoon dry oregano

Directions:

1. Season the chicken with salt and place it in a pan with heated olive oil.
2. Drizzle dried oregano and pepper over it and covered the chicken to cook for 10 minutes.
3. Flip the fillets and cook again for 10 minutes.
4. Whisk Dijon mustard, olive oil, balsamic, pepper, oregano and salt in a bowl.
5. Toss the chopped dried lettuce with the mustard vinaigrette.
6. Dice the chicken in cubes and serve it with lettuce, olives, and mushrooms.

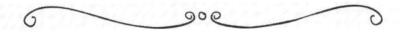

Moroccan Broccoli Chicken
Prep + Cook time: 35 minutes | Serves: 2

Nutritional Info (per serving)

Calories	Fat (g)	Protein (g)	Carbs (g)
267	9.3	32.2	14.8

Ingredients

2 chicken breast, pasture raised, cut inbite-size pieces

1 onion, cut in julienne

1 big garlic clove,smashed and finely chopped

zest from 1/2 lime

4 tbs. ras el hanout spice mix

few tbs. extra-virgin olive oil

1 bunch baby broccoli

1/4 cup slivered blanched almonds

10-15 leaves of fresh mint

1 tbs. arrowroot powder

salt to taste

water

Directions:

1. Dice the chicken into cubes and mix it with lime zest, olive oil, and Ras el hanout.
2. Marinate the chicken cubes for 20 minutes at room temperature.
3. Let your oven preheat at 350 degrees F.
4. Spread the sliced almonds in a baking sheet.
5. Toast the almonds in the oven for 8 minutes.
6. Take a sauté pan and add olive oil to heat.
7. Add onion and sauté until soft then add garlic and Ras el hanout.
8. Toss in the chicken and cook for 7 minutes.
9. Pour ½ cup water or stock along with some salt.
10. Add broccoli to the chicken and cover the pan.
11. Let it cook on a low simmer.
12. Mix 1 tbs. arrowroot in water and pour the mixture into the broccoli.
13. Stir cook for 30 seconds until it thickens.
14. Garnish with mint leaves and toasted almonds.
15. Enjoy.

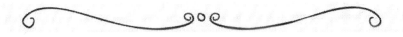

Chicken Pot Pie

Prep + Cook time: 55 minutes | Serves: 4

Nutritional Info (per serving)

Calories	*Fat (g)*	*Protein (g)*	*Carbs (g)*
584	42.7	25.8	26.7

Ingredients:

FOR THE CRUST:

1 cup almond flour

1/2 cup coconut flour

1/2 cup tapioca starch

1/2 cup cubed cold butter

1/2 teaspoon fine sea salt

1 whole pastured egg

½ cup Egg wash

FOR THE FILLING:

2 cups of chopped chicken

avocado oil

1 sweet onion, chopped finely

1 medium carrot, peeled and diced

½ lb. mix of mushrooms

1 bunch fresh parsley, chopped

1/2 bunch asparagus, chopped

1 cup chicken or vegetable broth

1/4 cup organic heavy cream

salt and pepper to taste

2 tbs. arrowroot powder

Directions:

1. Start by mixing ingredients for the crust in a processor.
2. Grind butter with salt and flour then beat in egg.
3. Once smooth, wrap the dough in a plastic sheet and refrigerate.
4. Season the chicken liberally with salt and pepper.
5. Sear it in a pan with heated avocado oil for 10 minutes.
6. Flip the chicken and cover it to cook more for 10 to 15 minutes.
7. Transfer the chicken meat to a bowl and set it aside.
8. Toss in the onion to the same pan with more oil. Sauté until soft.
9. Stir in carrots and mushrooms. Stir cook for 10 minutes.
10. Pour in chicken stock and cook it on a simmer for 5 minutes.
11. Add cream and cook more for 3 -5 minutes.
12. Return the chicken to the cooking pan then mix gently.
13. Mix arrowroot with water and pour this mixture into the chicken.
14. Cook until the mixture thickens then add parsley and asparagus. Turn off the heat.
15. Let your oven preheat 375 degrees F.
16. Divide the filling into two pie dishes.
17. Roll the refrigerated dough into two pie dish sized circles.
18. Place each circle on top of each dish.
19. Brush the top with egg wash liberally.
20. Bake them for 20 minutes until golden from the top.
21. Slice and enjoy.

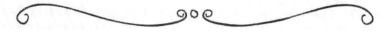

Orange Chicken with Brussel Sprouts

Prep + Cook time: 35 minutes | Serves: 4

Nutritional Info (per serving)

Calories	*Fat (g)*	*Protein (g)*	*Carbs (g)*
167	3.9	28.2	3.4

Ingredients:

FOR THE CHICKEN:

4 boneless pasture raised chicken thighs

Himalayan pink salt, to taste

fresh ground pepper, to taste

2 tbs. orange juice

2-3 orange wedges

avocado oil

FOR THE BRUSSEL SPROUTS:

1lbs brussels sprouts halved

salt and pepper

avocado oil

Directions:

1. Let your oven preheat at 375 degrees F.
2. Pat dry the chicken thighs then season it with all the spices.
3. Pour orange juice and avocado oil.
4. Place orange wedges over it then marinate for 20 minutes.

5. Toss sliced Brussel sprouts with avocado oil, salt, and pepper in a baking sheet.
6. Place the marinated chicken in the same sheet.
7. Bake them together for 20 minutes.
8. Turn the oven to broiler settings and broil for 5 minutes more.
9. Serve warm with cranberry sauce.
10. Enjoy.

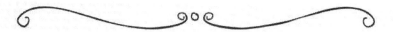

Sea Vegetables Chicken Salad
Prep + Cook time: 25 minutes | Serves: 4

Nutritional Info (per serving)

Calories	*Fat (g)*	*Protein (g)*	*Carbs (g)*
217	12.4	13.8	48.4

Ingredients:

1 pack Sea Tangle Mixed Sea Vegetables, rinsed and de-salted

1 pack Miracle Noodles Angel Hair

2, slices of cooked chicken breast

1 avocado, diced

2 cups of romaine lettuce, chopped

2 cups of baby spinach

FOR THE DRESSING:

1 garlic clove, grated

1-piece fresh ginger thumb size, grated

4 tbs. coconut aminos   salt and pepper to taste

4 tbs. apple cider vinegar

Directions:

1. Cook the noodles as per the pack's instructions then drain them.
2. Rinse and dry the seaweed as written on its packet.
3. Toss all the ingredients for dressing together in a bowl.
4. Divide the noodles into two serving bowls.
5. Top the noodles with all the solid ingredients.
6. Pour the prepared dressing on top.
7. Enjoy.

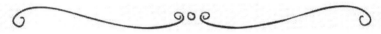

Creamy Mushroom Chicken
Prep + Cook time: 55 minutes | Serves: 4

Nutritional Info (per serving)

Calories	Fat (g)	Protein (g)	Carbs (g)
330	24.4	23.3	9.9

Ingredients:

To Make the Chicken Stock:

15-20 oz. pasture-raised chicken with bones

2 cups of mixed vegetables

Spices: 2 bay leaves, peppercorns, iodized sea salt

Creamy Mushroom and Chicken:

10 big cremini whole mushrooms, washed, dried and sliced

3 garlic cloves, peeled

1 sprig of thyme

1 bunch fresh parsley, washed, dried and chopped

1 can full-fat coconut milk

about 1 cup of chicken stock

2 tbs. arrowroot flour

avocado oil

salt and pepper to taste

lemon juice to taste

the cooked carrot if using

Directions:

1. Boil chicken in a stock pot half filled with water for 20 minutes.
2. Continue skimming off the fat from the top.
3. Add vegetables, bay leaves, peppercorns, and salt. Let it simmer more for 20 minutes.
4. Remove the carrot and chicken from the pot and place them in a plate.
5. Strain the remaining stock and discard all solids.
6. Shred the chicken meat after removing it from the bones.
7. Heat avocado oil in a large sauté pan.
8. Add mushrooms and garlic, sauté for 15 minutes.
9. Stir in shredded chicken then add coconut milk and 1 cup prepared stock.
10. First, boil then simmer it for 10 minutes.
11. Mix arrowroot with 1 tbs. water and pour it into the soup.
12. Stir cook for 5 minutes then add salt, pepper, lemon juice, and parsley.

13. Chop the carrots and add them to the soup.
14. Enjoy.

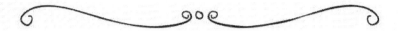

Spinach Stuffed Chicken Breast
Prep + Cook time: 35 minutes | Serves: 4

Nutritional Info (per serving)

Calories	Fat (g)	Protein (g)	Carbs (g)
323	13.2	43.8	8.1

Ingredients:

4 pasture raised chicken breasts

2 bunches of spinach

1 cup grated Pecorino Romano cheese

3 heaped tbs. avocado mayonnaise

2 teaspoon Italian herbs mix

1-2 teaspoon Hungarian paprika

1/4 teaspoon garlic powder

1 teaspoon oregano

salt and pepper

avocado oil

Directions:

1. Let your oven preheat at 375 degrees F.
2. Wash and drain the spinach then chop it finely.
3. Toss spinach with Romano and mayonnaise in a suitable bowl.

4. Place the chicken breasts on a working board and carve slit in the center horizontally from one side.
5. Once you get a pocket, rub it with salt, pepper, and herbs from inside.
6. Add spinach mixture to each pocket then seal it by inserting a toothpick.
7. Place the chicken in a baking sheet lined with wax paper.
8. Drizzle salt, pepper, paprika, garlic powder, oregano and avocado oil on top.
9. Bake, the chicken for 30 minutes in the preheated oven.
10. Switch the oven to broiler setting and bake more for 5 minutes.
11. Serve warm.

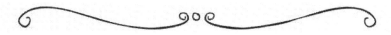

Chicken Schnitzel
Prep + Cook time: 25 minutes | Serves: 1

Nutritional Info (per serving)

Calories	Fat (g)	Protein (g)	Carbs (g)
375	10.7	35.1	30.5

Ingredients:

1 pasture raised chicken breast

1 pastured egg

5 tbs. almond flour

3 tbs. cassava flour

avocado oil for frying

salt and pepper to taste

other chicken spices, optional

Directions:

1. Cut the chicken into 2 equally thick slices and pound them with a mallet.
2. Season each with salt and pepper liberally.
3. Whisk 1 egg with salt and pepper in a shallow plate.
4. Toss all the flours with salt and pepper in another shallow plate.
5. Preheat a pan with avocado oil on medium heat.
6. Dredge the chicken pieces in the dry flour mixture then dip in the eggs.
7. Repeat the dredging and dipping then place the slices in the pan.
8. Cook them until they are golden brown from each side.
9. Serve warm.

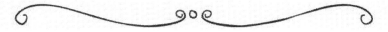

Mustard Chicken Wings
Prep + Cook time: 1hr. 15 minutes | Serves: 4

Nutritional Info (per serving)

Calories	Fat (g)	Protein (g)	Carbs (g)
450	8.8	67.1	21.7

Ingredients:

For Chicken Wings

2 lbs. pasture raised chicken wings

Dry spice mix: sage, thyme, yellow mustard, black pepper, coarse salt, garlic powder

Avocado oil

FOR SWEET POTATOE FRIES

2 sweet potatoes, cut into French fried shaped slices

Dry spice mix: sage, thyme, yellow mustard, black pepper, coarse salt

1 teaspoon arrowroot powder

Avocado oil

Directions:

1. Let your oven preheat at 375 degrees F.
2. Pat dry the chicken wings then season liberally with spice mixture.
3. Drizzle 1 tbs. avocado oil and rub it well too.
4. Place the wings in a baking pan and bake them for 30 minutes.
5. Meanwhile, prepare the potato fries. Spread the sliced potatoes in a baking sheet.
6. Toss the potatoes with spices, 1 teaspoon avocado oil, and arrowroot starch.
7. Once the chicken is done, switch the oven to 425 degrees F.
8. Flip the wings and place potatoes in the next rack in the oven.
9. Bake again for 30 minutes. Flip the wings halfway through.
10. Drizzle the malt vinegar over the wings.
11. Serve warm.

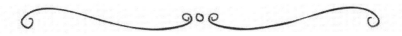

Chicken Salad Nori Rolls

Prep + Cook time: 15 minutes | Serves: 2

Nutritional Info (per serving)

Calories	*Fat (g)*	*Protein (g)*	*Carbs (g)*
83	1.5	9	7

Ingredients:

For the Rolls:

1 pack Organic Miracle Rice

3 roasted Nori sheets

1 cup of home-made chicken salad

few handfuls of baby arugula

For Serving:

red radishes, finely sliced

pickled ginger

wasabi pastes

Hot sauce

Coconut aminos

Directions:

1. Prepare the rice as per the given instructions on its packet.
2. Mix 2 tbs. wasabi powder with water to make a thick paste.

3. Spread the nori sheet on a bamboo sheet as you prepare the filling.
4. Spread the layer of prepare rice, then top it with chicken.
5. Start rolling the nori sheet into a sushi roll.
6. Slice the roll into thick pieces.
7. Serve them with wasabi paste and other toppings.
8. Enjoy.

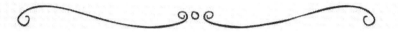

Tarragon Chicken Salad with Cranberries
Prep + Cook time: 35 minutes | Serves: 2

Nutritional Info (per serving)

Calories	Fat (g)	Protein (g)	Carbs (g)
154	3	28	2.2

Ingredients:

2 pasture raised chicken breasts

2 tbs. avocado oil

Salt and black pepper, to taste

2-3 stacks celery, finely chopped

a handful of unsweetened dry cranberries

2 stems of fresh tarragon

1/2 cup avocado mayonnaise

1/4 lemon, juice

salt and pepper to taste

Directions:

1. Let your oven preheat at 370 degrees F.

2. Place the chicken breasts in a pan and rub them with salt, pepper and avocado oil.
3. Place lemon slices on top then cover the pan with a loose tent of aluminum foil.
4. Bake the chicken for 30 minutes.
5. Allow the cooked chicken to cool then chop it into pieces.
6. Toss the chopped celery with tarragon and cranberries in a bowl.
7. Add chicken, olive oil, salt, pepper, lemon juice, and mayonnaise.
8. Serve fresh.

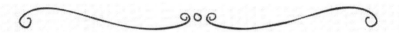

Flat Chicken Nuggets

Prep + Cook time: 25 minutes | Serves: 2

Nutritional Info (per serving)

Calories	Fat (g)	Protein (g)	Carbs (g)
301	12.3	35.8	9.4

Ingredients:

2 chicken breasts (halves) from a pasture raised chicken

2 pasture raised eggs

Spices:

iodized sea

salt, pepper,

2/3 cup almond flour

1/2 cup cassava flour

Avocado oil

Hungarian paprika,

organic garlic and onion
powders

Directions:

1. Let your oven preheat at 400 degrees F.
2. Slice the chicken into strips and season liberally with all the spices.
3. Spread the two flours in two different plates.
4. Beat eggs with salt and pepper in another shallow plate.
5. Dredge the strips first through cassava flour then dip into the egg mixture.
6. Now coat then stripes with almond flour.
7. Place the strips in a baking pan greased with avocado oil.
8. Bake them for 20 minutes.
9. Serve warm.

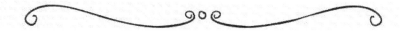

Chicken Ramen Soup
Prep + Cook time: 25 minutes | Serves: 2

Nutritional Info (per serving)

Calories	*Fat (g)*	*Protein (g)*	*Carbs (g)*
191	4.1	23.8	14.3

Ingredients:

28 oz. chicken stock

1 bag of Miracle Noodle capellini

2 tbs. Miso Paste

about 6 oz. cooked chicken breast, sliced

1 cup shredded green cabbage	1 small raw carrot, peeled and ribboned
2 bok choy, cut in half	few scallions
handful of cilantro	pepper and salt, to taste

Directions:

1. Cook the noodles as per the given instructions on the packet. Drain and set aside.
2. Heat the stock in the soup pot and stir in cabbage.
3. Boil it in 7 minutes then add chicken and bok choy.
4. Let it simmer in 4 minutes then turn off the heat.
5. Add miso paste and mix well.
6. Divide the noodles and soup into the serving bowls.
7. Garnish with scallions, cilantro and carrot ribbons.
8. Enjoy.

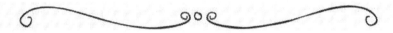

Aji de Gallina
Prep + Cook time: 55 minutes | Serves: 4

Nutritional Info (per serving)

Calories	*Fat (g)*	*Protein (g)*	*Carbs (g)*
574	34.2	41	30.7

Ingredients:

For the Chicken Stock:

2 lbs. chicken with bones	2 big stalks celery
1 yellow onion	1 carrot

1 parsnip

For the Dish:

2 cups shredded chicken

1 cup chicken stock

1 can full coconut milk

1/2 cup walnuts

1/2 cup grated Parmigiano Reggiano

2 tbs. Cassava Flour

1 big yellow onion, chopped

2 big garlic cloves, smashed and chopped

2 tbs. avocado oil

1 teaspoon red chili paste

2 tbs. Smoked Jalapeno Sriracha

2 tbs. turmeric powder

salt and pepper to taste

kalamata olives

2 hard-boiled eggs

3-4 bags of miracle rice

Directions:

1. Boil chicken and vegetables in water in 40 minutes to make the stock.
2. Once done, strain the stock and keep the chicken aside.
3. Discard all the solids. Remove the chicken meat from the bones.
4. Shred the chicken and keep it aside.
5. Hard boil two pastured eggs then peel them.
6. Now cook the miracle rice as per the given instructions on the packet.
7. Drain and fry the rice and keep them aside.
8. Sauté chopped onions and garlic in heated avocado oil for 5 minutes.
9. Meanwhile blend coconut milk with walnuts, cassava flour, parmesan, and stock.

10. Add chicken shreds, coconut milk mixture and chili paste to the pan.
11. Boil the mixture then add turmeric, salt, and pepper.
12. Serve with parsley, miracle rice, olives, and boiled egg slices.

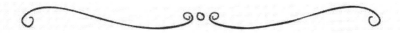

Lemon Garlic Chicken
Prep + Cook time: 15 minutes | Serves: 2

Nutritional Info (per serving)

Calories	*Fat (g)*	*Protein (g)*	*Carbs (g)*
246	9.7	29.9	8.4

Ingredients:

1–2 pounds chicken breasts or thighs

1 onion, diced

1 tbs. avocado oil, lard, or ghee

1 teaspoon of salt

5 garlic cloves, minced

1/2 cup organic chicken broth

1 teaspoon dried parsley

1/4 teaspoon paprika

1/4 cup white cooking wine

1 large lemon juiced

3–4 teaspoons arrowroot flour

Directions:

1. Select Sauté on your Instant pot and sauté onion in some oil until soft.

2. Stir in all the remaining ingredients except arrowroot flour.
3. Seal the lid and select Poultry mode. Seal the pressure valve.
4. Once done, release the steam completely then from the lid.
5. Mix arrowroot flour with ¼ cup of the cooking liquid.
6. Pour this slurry into the pot.
7. Mix well and cook on Sauté mode for 2 minutes.
8. Serve warm.

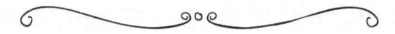

Lemongrass Coconut Chicken
Prep + Cook time: 25 minutes | Serves: 4

Nutritional Info (per serving)

Calories	Fat (g)	Protein (g)	Carbs (g)
578	31.2	60.5	7.5

Ingredients:

1 thick stalk fresh lemongrass, trimmed

4 cloves garlic, peeled and minced

1 thumb-size piece of ginger, peeled and minced

2 tbs. Red Boat fish sauce

3 tbs. coconut aminos

1 teaspoon five spice powder

1 cup full-fat coconut milk

10 drumsticks, skin removed

1 teaspoon kosher salt

½ teaspoon freshly ground black pepper

1 teaspoon coconut oil

1 large onion, peeled and thinly sliced

¼ cup fresh cilantro, chopped

Juice from 1 lime (optional)

Directions:

1. Blend lemongrass with fish sauce, garlic, ginger, coconut aminos, five spice in a blender.
2. Add coconut milk and blend again to form a sauce.
3. Pat dry the drumsticks and season them with salt and pepper.
4. Select Sauté on your Instant pot and sauté onion with 1 teaspoon oil in it.
5. After 3 minutes add chicken and pour the lemongrass sauce on top.
6. Secure the lid of the cooker and turn the pressure release handle to theclosed position.
7. Select Manual mode with high pressure and 15 minutes of cooking time.
8. Once done, release the pressure completely then remove the lid.
9. Adjust seasoning with salt and pepper.
10. Enjoy.

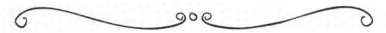

Chicken Paprikash Hungarian Stew
Prep + Cook time: 25 minutes | Serves: 4

Nutritional Info (per serving)

Calories	Fat (g)	Protein (g)	Carbs (g)
418	22.6	47.2	10.2

Ingredients:

2 lbs. chicken leg quarters or drumsticks

1 tbs olive oil

1 medium onion, thinly sliced

3 cloves garlic, minced

½ medium zucchini, chopped

3 tbs paprika

1/2 cup chicken stock

1 tbs. arrowroot or arrowroot powder

1 tbs fresh lemon juice

1/2 cup sour cream

1 tbs parsley, chopped

salt and pepper, to taste

Directions:

1. Select Sauté on your Instant pot and heat 1 tbs. olive oil in it.
2. Season meat pieces liberally with salt and pepper.
3. Sear it in the oil for 3 mins per side.
4. Dish out the chicken to a plate and keep it aside.
5. Add garlic and onions to the pot and sauté them for 2 mins.
6. Toss in zucchini and cook for 2 minutes.
7. Add paprika, salt, broth,and chicken to the pot.
8. Secure the lid and select Manual mode with high settings for 10 minutes.
9. Once done, release the pressure completely then remove the lid.
10. Mix ¼ cup of cooking liquid with arrowroot in a bowl.
11. Add this slurry to the chicken and cook on sauté mode for 2 minutes.
12. Stir in lemon juice, sour cream, and parsley.
13. Enjoy.

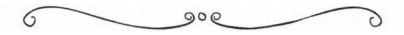

Easy Sweet Chicken

Prep + Cook time: 50 minutes | Serves: 3

Nutritional Info (per serving)

Calories	*Fat (g)*	*Protein (g)*	*Carbs (g)*
653	10.5	41.8	104

Ingredients:

3 lbs. chicken breasts or chicken tenders

1 cup honey

1/2 cup ketchup

1/2 cup gluten-free soy sauce

2 cloves garlic, minced

Directions:

1. Spread a layer of aluminum foil in a 9x13 inch baking pan.
2. Place the chicken in the baking pan.
3. Whisk all the remaining ingredients and pour the mixture over the chicken.
4. Bake it for 45 minutes in a preheated oven at 375 degrees F.
5. Once done, serve warm as desired.

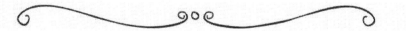

Hawaiian Chicken

Prep + Cook time: 25 minutes | Serves: 4

Calories	Fat (g)	Protein (g)	Carbs (g)
125	1.3	10.9	18.2

Ingredients:

1/4 cup lectin free soy sauce

1 tbs. garlic, diced

1/4 cup raw honey

2 large chicken breasts

Directions:

1. Mix honey with soy sauce and garlic in a bowl.
2. Heat this mixture in the microwave for 30 seconds on low temperature.
3. Place chicken in a ziplock pouch and pour the garlic marinade in it.
4. Seal the chicken and shake the bag to coat the chicken well.
5. Let the chicken marinate for 1 hour in the refrigerator.
6. During this preheat the oven at 375 degrees F.
7. Arrange the chicken in a baking tray and bake for 20 minutes more until al dente.
8. Enjoy.

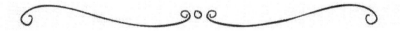

Rotisserie Spice Chicken

Prep + Cook time: 45 minutes | Serves: 6

Nutritional Info (per serving)

Calories	Fat (g)	Protein (g)	Carbs (g)

588	37.9	56.8	5.9

Ingredients:

Whole Chicken, 3-4lbs

2 teaspoons Paprika

2 teaspoon garlic powder

1 1/2 teaspoon Kosher salt

1 1/2 teaspoon Onion powder

1/4 teaspoon Turmeric

1/4 teaspoon ground pepper

1/2 teaspoon Dried Thyme

1 tbs. avocado oil

1 medium white onion

1 stalk celery

1 lemon, cut in half and seeded

1/2 cup chicken stock or water

1 tbs arrowroot powder

Directions:

1. Clean the chicken from inside then rinse it well. Pat dry it well with paper towel.
2. Combine all the spices with 1 tbs. oil to make a paste.
3. Brush the chicken with this spice mixture then place it in the Instant Pot.
4. Select Sauté and sear it for 4 minutes.
5. Flip the chicken and cook for another 4 minutes.
6. Add chicken stock, broth, half onion sliced.
7. Stuff the seared chicken with lemon slices, whole onion, and celery.
8. Return the chicken to the pot and Secure the lid.
9. Select Manual function for 25 minutes at high pressure.
10. Once done, remove the pressure completely.
11. Transfer the chicken to the serving plate.
12. Mix arrowroot with ¼ cup cooking liquid and pour it into the pot.

13. Cook on sauté mode until it thickens. Pour the sauce over the chicken.
14. Enjoy.

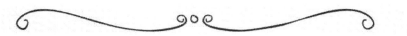

Chicken Ponzu Stir-Fry
Prep + Cook time: 25 minutes | Serves: 2

Nutritional Info (per serving)

Calories	*Fat (g)*	*Protein (g)*	*Carbs (g)*
243	3.7	25.8	27.1

Ingredients:

1⅛ lbs. chopped Chicken Breast

6 oz. Carrots

15 oz.baby Bok Choy

½ cup Asian-Style Sautéed Aromatics

¼ cup spicy Ponzu Sauce

2 Tbs. Hoisin Sauce

2 Tbs. Black Bean Sauce

Directions:

1. Combine black bean sauce with hoisin, ponzu sauce along with aromatics.
2. Pat dry the chicken paper towel then rub it with salt, pepper, and arrowroot.
3. Preheat 2 ½ tbs. oil in ant cooking pot and add chicken and carrots.
4. Stir cook for 4 minutes until brown.

5. Toss bok choy and prepared sauce along with salt and pepper.
6. Stir cook for 5 minutes.
7. Serve warm with cook rice.

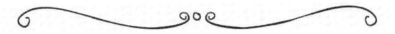

Stir-Fried Curry Chicken
Prep + Cook time: 35 minutes | Serves: 2

Nutritional Info (per serving)

Calories	Fat (g)	Protein (g)	Carbs (g)
726	51.1	21	53.4

Ingredients:

1⅛ lbs. Chopped Chicken Breast

1 cup Jasmine Rice

1¾ cups Light Coconut Milk

1 Yellow Onion

10 oz. Baby Bok Choy

2 cloves Garlic

2 oz. Sliced Roasted Red Peppers, peeled and deseeded

2 Tbs. Crème Fraiche

2 teaspoon Vadouvan Curry Powder

Directions:

1. Mix rice with coconut milk, ¾ cup water and a pinch of salt in a pot.
2. Cook the rice for 20 minutes until al dente then keep them aside.
3. Toss onion with garlic in a bowl.

4. Pat dry the chicken and season it liberally with curry powder, salt, and pepper.
5. Heat 2 tbs. olive oil in a suitable pan.
6. Cook chicken in the heated oil for 3 minutes then add garlic and onion.
7. Sauté for 6 minutes then add pepper, and crème fraiche
8. Serve warm.

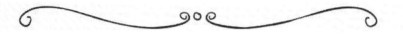

Spicy Glazed Chicken
Prep + Cook time: 35 minutes | Serves: 4

Nutritional Info (per serving)

Calories	*Fat (g)*	*Protein (g)*	*Carbs (g)*
296	3.2	53.8	12.5

Ingredients:

2 Boneless, Skinless Chicken Breasts

6 oz. Carrots, chopped

10 oz. Baby Bok Choy, diced

2 cloves Garlic, minced

3 oz. Radishes, grated

2 teaspoon Gochujang

1 Tbs. Honey

1 Tbs. Rice Vinegar

Directions:

1. Combine honey with ¼ cup water, salt, pepper and gochujang in a bowl.
2. Mix radishes with 1 teaspoon olive oil, salt, pepper, and vinegar in another bowl.

3. Let it marinate for 10 minutes with occasional stirring.
4. Meanwhile, preheat 2 teaspoons olive oil in a medium pan.
5. Add bok choy stems, salt, pepper, and carrots. Sauté for 3 minutes.
6. Add bok choy leaves, and garlic then sauté for 2 minutes.
7. Transfer the mix to a bowl and keep it warm.
8. Pat dry the meatwith a paper towel then season it with salt and pepper.
9. Cook the seasoned chicken in 2 teaspoons olive oil on medium heat for 4 minutes per side.
10. Add the honey glaze and mix gently.
11. Toss in the cooked vegetables.
12. Serve warm with marinated radishes.

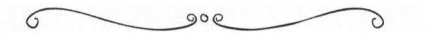

Coq Au Vin
Prep + Cook time: 45 minutes | Serves: 4

Nutritional Info (per serving)

Calories	*Fat (g)*	*Protein (g)*	*Carbs (g)*
649	22.7	63.8	22.4

Ingredients:

2 cups red wine

1 cup chopped yellow onion

1 cup chopped carrot

1 teaspoon salt

1 teaspoon dried thyme

1/2 teaspoon dried rosemary, crushed

1/2 teaspoon freshly ground black pepper

2 (8-ounce) chicken breast halves, skinned

2 (4-ounce) chicken thighs, skinned

2 (4-ounce) chicken drumsticks, skinned

1/2 cup all-purpose flour

3 bacon slices, chopped

1/2 cup pitted dried plums, quartered

2 bay leaves

Chopped fresh parsley (optional)

Directions:

1. Toss red wine, onion, carrot, salt, dried thyme, dried rosemary, black pepper, chicken thighs and drumsticks in a large bowl.
2. Cover this chicken and marinate for 4 hours in the refrigerator.
3. Remove the chicken from the marinade then pat it dry.
4. Spread flour in a shallow dish and coat the chicken in this flour.
5. Sauté bacon in a Dutch oven until crispy then transfer it to a plate.
6. Add chicken in batches and cook it well until golden brown.
7. Add carrot, and onion from the marinade and sauté for 5 minutes.
8. Stir in bacon, plums, and leaves.
9. Cook this mixture on medium high heat for 30 minutes until chicken is done.
10. Discard bay leaves and enjoy with parsley leaves on top.

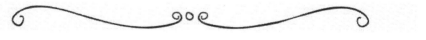

Chicken Parmesan

Prep + Cook time: 25 minutes | Serves: 2

Nutritional Info (per serving)

Calories	*Fat (g)*	*Protein (g)*	*Carbs (g)*
355	32.6	14.9	2.5

Ingredients:

1/4 cup almond flour
Salt and pepper, to taste
1 1/3 pounds chicken cutlets
1 1/2 tbs. olive oil
1/2 cup dry red
1 1/2 cups tomato sauce

4 ounces skim mozzarella, shredded
2 tbs. parsley, chopped
1 tbs. Parmesan cheese, finely grated, for serving

Directions:

1. Toss flour with salt and pepper and add it to a Ziplock pouch.
2. Place chicken in the bag and shake it well to coat.
3. Heat oil in a suitably sized pan and sear the coated chicken well in 4 minutes.
4. Transfer the chicken to a plate.
5. Add wine to the pan and stir cook for 2 minutes
6. Then add tomato sauce and the chicken. Cook for 3 minutes.
7. Add mozzarella and parsley.
8. Garnish with parmesan.
9. Enjoy.

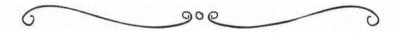

Garlic Roast Chicken
Prep + Cook time: 1hr. 35 minutes | Serves: 8

Nutritional Info (per serving)

Calories	Fat (g)	Protein (g)	Carbs (g)
739	52.9	64.4	3.4

Ingredients:

1 (6-to 7-pounds) whole roasting chicken, giblets removed

9 sprigs fresh thyme

9 sprigs fresh tarragon

1 lemon, halved

4 heads garlic, cloves separated, unpeeled

1 cup Niçoise olives

1 teaspoon coarse salt

1/2 teaspoon freshly ground black pepper

1/3 cup extra-virgin olive oil

1 large baguette, thickly sliced

Directions:

1. Let your oven preheat at 450 degrees F.
2. Loose up the chicken skin and stuff it with 1/3 of thyme and tarragon.
3. Add the 1/3 of herbs, garlic cloves, and lemon to the chicken cavity.
4. Tie the chicken legs with butcher thread.
5. Keep the chicken in a roasting pan and spread herbs, olives, and garlic on top.
6. Drizzle salt, pepper, and olive oil.
7. Bake the chicken for 1.5 hours in the preheated oven.
8. Serve warm.

Sesame Chicken Salad

Prep + Cook time: 20 minutes | Serves: 2

Nutritional Info (per serving)

Calories	*Fat (g)*	*Protein (g)*	*Carbs (g)*
410	11.1	35.6	43.9

Ingredients:

10 oz. Chopped Chicken Breast

½ lb. Cabbage, sliced

6 oz. Carrots, diced

2 cloves Garlic, minced

1 bunch Mint, chopped

1 Tbs. Sambal Oelek

1 Tbs. Sesame Oil

1 Tbs. Soy Sauce

1 Tbs. Rice Vinegar

1 Tbs. Honey

Directions:

1. Season the chicken with salt and pepper.
2. Preheat sesame oil in a pan and place the seasoned chicken in it.
3. Cook for 2-3 minutes per side then add half of the soy sauce and garlic.
4. Stir cook for 4 minutes then turn off the heat.
5. Mix honey with vinegar, soy sauce, Sambal Oelek, sesame oil, salt and pepper in a bowl.
6. Toss all the vegetables, cooked chicken and Oelek dressing in a bowl.
7. Garnish with mint and enjoy.

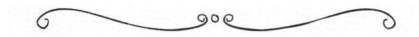

Chicken with Dumplings

Prep + Cook time: 45 minutes | Serves: 6

Nutritional Info (per serving)

Calories	*Fat (g)*	*Protein (g)*	*Carbs (g)*
663	25.5	90.4	11.6

Ingredients:

Cooking spray

1 cup chopped onion

1 garlic clove, chopped

1/4 cup dry sherry

1/2 teaspoon salt

1/4 teaspoon black pepper

2 (14 1/2-ounce) cans fat-free, less-sodium chicken broth

1 (10 3/4-ounce) can condensed cream of mushroom soup, undiluted

4 pounds chicken pieces, skinned

1 cup of frozen green peas

1/4 cup water

2 tbs. arrowroot powder

6 precooked almond flour dumplings

Chopped parsley (optional)

Directions:

1. Heat a greased Dutch oven and sauté onion and garlic in it, for 5 minutes.
2. Toss in chicken pieces along with sherry, broth, salt, and pepper.

3. After boiling the mixture, reduce it to simmer and cook for 35 minutes.
4. Transfer the chicken to a suitable bowl using a slotted spoon.
5. Remove the meat from the bones and dice it into chunks.
6. Return the meat along with peas to the Dutch oven.
7. Mix arrowroot powder with 2 tbs. water and pour it into the chicken.
8. Add almond flour dumplings.
9. Garnish with parsley.
10. Serve warm.

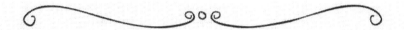

Beef, Pork & Lamb Recipes

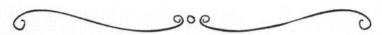

Spinach Meatloaf

Prep + Cook time: 55 minutes | Serves: 4

Nutritional Info (per serving)

Calories	*Fat (g)*	*Protein (g)*	*Carbs (g)*
456	12.7	28.1	54.3

Ingredients:

1 medium yellow onion, finely chopped

2 big stalks celery, finely chopped

1 small carrot or parsnip, grated

1 small sweet potato, peeled and grated

1 bunch spinach

1 lb. grass fed ground beef

1 pastured egg

6 tbs. cassava flour

2 tbs. dry parsley, chopped

1 tbs. dry oregano

1/2 tbs. dry thyme

1 teaspoon salt

1 teaspoon pepper

avocado oil

Directions:

1. Let your oven preheat at 350 degrees F.
2. Line three small loaf pans with parchment paper.
3. Preheat avocado oil in a pan. Sauté celery and onion for 7 minutes in it.
4. Stir in spinach and cook for 4 minutes.
5. Add meat mince, sweet potato, parsnip, and carrot. Add 1 teaspoon water to the mixture.
6. Mix this mixture well then divide the mixture in the loaf pans.

7. Bake them for 45 minutes then allow the loaf to cool for 10 minutes.

8. Slice and serve.

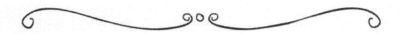

Broccoli and Beef Stir Fry
Prep + Cook time: 35 minutes | Serves: 4

Nutritional Info (per serving)

Calories	Fat (g)	Protein (g)	Carbs (g)
450	27.9	37.8	13.1

Ingredients:

1 lb. beef sirloin steak, boneless ribeye steak

1 lb. broccoli florets

baking soda

1/4 cup coconut aminos

2 tbs. fresh lime juice

1/2 teaspoon garlic powder

1/4 cup lard/tallow/coconut oil

1/4 teaspoon pure stevia extract

1 t. fresh minced ginger

2 tbs. Oil for the frying pan

Xanthan gum

Directions:

1. Slice the beef in the thin strip then coat the beef with baking soda.

2. Combine all the remaining ingredients except the broccoli, beef and xanthan gum.

3. Pour this marinade over the coated beef and let it marinate for 20 minutes.
4. Steam the broccoli florets over boiling water until they are soft.
5. Drain and allow the broccoli florets to cool.
6. Pour the 2 tbs. oil in a skillet and preheat it.
7. Stir in meat and cook for 4-5 minutes until brown.
8. Toss in broccoli and xanthan gum.
9. Stir cook until it thickens.
10. Enjoy warm.

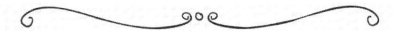

Winter Steak
Prep + Cook time: 15 minutes | Serves: 1

Nutritional Info (per serving)

Calories	Fat (g)	Protein (g)	Carbs (g)
572	59	12.9	1.7

Ingredients:

½ pound grass-fed steak,

¼ cup of coconut oil

1 teaspoon Real salt

½ teaspoon fresh ground black pepper

½ teaspoon garlic powder

Directions:

1. Pat dry the steaks using a paper towel.
2. Let your oven preheat at broiler settings.
3. Preheat coconut oil in a cast iron pan.
4. Season the steaks with garlic, pepper, and salt.

5. Add the garlic steaks to the pan and sear the steak for 1 minute per side.

6. Place the pan inthe broiler and broil it for 2 minutes.

7. Serve warm.

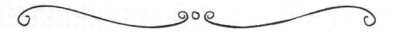

Italian Mushroom Roast
Prep + Cook time: 45 minutes | Serves: 4

Nutritional Info (per serving)

Calories	*Fat (g)*	*Protein (g)*	*Carbs (g)*
362	11.3	54.5	8.2

Ingredients

1 1/4 teaspoon dried Italian seasoning

1 1/2 lbs. boneless beef chuck roast, cut into 4 chunks

10 oz. white mushrooms, diced

1/2 teaspoon sea salt

1 medium sweet onion, sliced

1 small zucchini, thinelysliced

1/4 teaspoon fresh ground black pepper

Au Jus

2 tbs. red wine vinegar

1/3 cup beef or chicken stock

1 tbs. Worcestershire sauce

Directions:

1. Grease a pressure cooker with coconut oil.
2. Season the roast with seasonings and place it in the cooker.
3. Top the roast with onion, zucchini, and mushrooms.
4. Mix vinegar and Worcestershire sauce, pour this sauce in the cooker.
5. Secure the lid and select 'Manual' mode at high pressure for 25 minutes.
6. Once done, release the pressure completely then remove the lid.
7. Stir well and garnish as desired.
8. Serve warm.

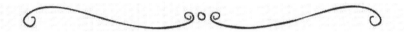

Rib Roast with Caramelized Onions
Prep + Cook time: 55 minutes | Serves: 6

Nutritional Info (per serving)

Calories	*Fat (g)*	*Protein (g)*	*Carbs (g)*
370	17.7	31.4	9.9

Ingredients:

3 lb. cross rib roast

2 cups red wine or kombucha

1/4 cup Bragg's liquid aminos

3 tbs. olive oil

1 onion, diced or chopped the way you like them

6-8 carrots, chopped

| 2-3 teaspoons garlic, minced | basil, oregano, kosher salt & pepper, to taste |

Directions:

1. Mix kombucha and aminos in a Ziplock bag.
2. Place the roast in this bag and seal it. shake well then marinate for 2 hrs.
3. Preheat olive oil in pressure cooker on 'Sauté' mode.
4. Add onions and sauté for 15 minutes then add marinated roast.
5. Toss in carrots then secure the lid.
6. Select 'Manual' function at high pressure for 45 minutes until roast is done.
7. Once done, release the pressure completely remove the lid.
8. Garnish it with spices and herbs.
9. Enjoy warm.

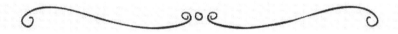

Cuban Beef
Prep + Cook time: 55 minutes | Serves: 4

Nutritional Info (per serving)

Calories	*Fat (g)*	*Protein (g)*	*Carbs (g)*
219	13.1	15.8	9.9

Ingredients:

| 2 tbs. coconut oil | 2 medium onions, sliced |
| 1 (2-3-pounds) bone-in chuck or arm roast | 1 medium carrot, roughly chopped |

1 celery stalk, roughly chopped

1 bay leaf

3 garlic cloves, 1 peeled and crushed and two diced

1-2 cups beef broth

2 teaspoons ground cumin

½ teaspoon cayenne

½ zucchini, chopped

½ teaspoon dried oregano

salt and pepper to taste

Directions:

1. Season the beef with pepper and salt liberally.
2. Preheat coconut oil in a pressure cooker on medium heat then sear the beef in it.
3. Once seared, transfer the beef to a plate.
4. Toss in carrot, celery, zucchini and onion, sauté until soft.
5. Stir in bay leaf and garlic, stir cook for 1 minute.
6. Add roast to the mixture along with broth and secure its lid.
7. Select 'Manual' function for 35 minutes at high pressure.
8. Once done, release the pressure completely then remove the lid.
9. Remove the meat from its cooker and allow it to cool
10. Strain the remaining cooking liquid and discard all solids.
11. Preheat coconut oil in a separate pot and sauté onion in it until soft.
12. Add cayenne, cumin, garlic, and stir cook for 2 minutes.
13. Pour in cooking liquid, salt, pepper, and oregano.
14. Let it cook for 15 minutes on a simmer.
15. Shred the cooked beef and add it to the cooking mixture.
16. Serve warm.

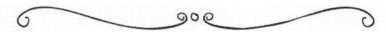

Lectin-Free Chili
Prep + Cook time: 35 minutes | Serves: 4

Nutritional Info (per serving)

Calories	Fat (g)	Protein (g)	Carbs (g)
570	38	50	6.7

Ingredients:

1 tbs. avocado oil, divided

2 pounds grass-fed ground beef

sea salt and black pepper

4 cloves garlic, minced

1 medium onion, finely diced

3 ribs celery, finely diced

2 tbs. chili powder

2 teaspoons ground cumin

1/4 teaspoon ground cinnamon

pinch ground cloves

2 cups grass-fed beef broth

3 ounces pine nuts

1 15-ounce can sweet potato purée

1 tbs. sauce from preserved chipotles in adobo

2 teaspoons red wine vinegar

2 teaspoons coconut aminos

sliced scallions and lime wedges, for garnish

sour cream, for serving (optional)

Directions:

1. Preheat a teaspoon of oil in a large skillet and stir fry ground beef with salt for 4 minutes.
2. Transfer this beef mince to the Instant Pot.
3. Add onion, celery, and garlic to the same skillet and sauté for 5 minutes.
4. Stir in cumin, cinnamon, chili powder, and cloves, then stir cook for 1 minute.

5. Pour in broth then transfer the mixture to the Instant Pot.
6. Add remaining ingredients to the Instant Pot and secure the lid.
7. Select Manual function, for 20 minutes at high pressure.
8. Once done, release the pressure completely.
9. Garnish with lime wedges, sour cream, and scallions.
10. Enjoy warm.

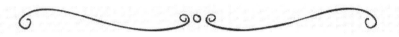

Shredded Beef
Prep + Cook time: 25 minutes | Serves: 6

Nutritional Info (per serving)

Calories	*Fat (g)*	*Protein (g)*	*Carbs (g)*
281	12.8	39	0.3

Ingredients:

3-4 lbs.of beef rump roast

2 tbs.avocado oil

1 teaspoon of sea salt

2 1/2 cups of bone broth

Directions:

1. Slice the roast into 4 equal size pieces and season them with salt.
2. Select Sauté function on Instant Pot and heat oil in its pot.
3. Add the beef and sear it well in 10 minutes.
4. Pour in broth and secure the lid.
5. Once done, release the pressure completely then remove the lid.

6. Transfer the meat to the working board and shred the meat using a fork.
7. Use this meat to stuff the gluten-free tortilla.
8. Serve.

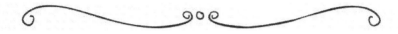

Pot Roast & Gravy

Prep + Cook time: 1hr. 20 minutes | Serves: 6

Nutritional Info (per serving)

Calories	*Fat (g)*	*Protein (g)*	*Carbs (g)*
752	26.3	103.9	20

Ingredients:

4 pounds chuck roast, diced into 4 chunks

a good pinch of salt

freshly ground black pepper

1 1/2 cups beef broth

2 tbs. balsamic vinegar

2 teaspoons fish sauce

1 three-inch sprig rosemary

4 three-inch sprigs thyme, whole

2 parsnips, peeled

4 carrots, peeled or scrubbed

6 cloves garlic, peeled

chopped parsley and/or chives for serving, optional

Directions:

1. Mix beef with salt and pepper to the pressure cooker.
2. Stir in all the remaining ingredients and secure the lid.
3. Select the Manual function at high pressure for 60 minutes.

4. Once done, release the pressure completely in 15 minutes.
5. Transfer the cooked meat to any plate and vegetable to a blender.
6. Discard the thyme and rosemary, preserve the cooking liquid.
7. Skim off the fats from the liquid surface then pour it into the blender.
8. Blend the veggies until smooth and season it with salt and pepper.
9. Shred the cooked meat using forks.
10. Heat the blended veggies mixture and add meat to the mixture.
11. Serve as desired.

Pork Loin with Creamy Gravy
Prep + Cook time: 45 minutes | Serves: 6

Nutritional Info (per serving)

Calories	Fat (g)	Protein (g)	Carbs (g)
810	52.8	65.5	17.3

Ingredients:

3lbs. Pork Loin

1 medium white onion, sliced

1lb carrots (about 4 medium sizes), chopped

2 avocado oil

1/2 teaspoon kosher salt

1 teaspoon garlic powder

1/2 teaspoon caraway seeds

1/2 teaspoon thyme

1/2 teaspoon paprika

1/2 teaspoon ground black pepper

1/4 cup water

Sour Cream Gravy Ingredients:

1 cup sour cream

1 Tbs. capers (or more to taste)

1/2 cup parsley

1 teaspoon caraway seeds

1 Tbs. arrowroot powder

1/2 teaspoon salt

Directions:

1. Select Sauté function on Instant pot and heat oil in it.
2. Season the pork loin with spices and sear it in the heated oil for 3 minutes until brown.
3. Transfer the pork to a plate then and carrots and onion.
4. Sauté them for 3 minutes then add ¼ cup water to deglaze the pot.
5. Return the pork to the pot and secure the lid.
6. Select Manual function for 20 minutes at high pressure.
7. Once done, release the pressure completely then remove the lid.
8. Transfer the pork to a working board and allow it to cool.
9. Keep 1/3 cup of cooking liquid in the Instant Pot and remove the remaining.
10. Add capers, parsley, arrowroot, sour cream and caraway seeds to the pot.
11. Puree this mixture using an immersion blender.
12. Cook this mixture on sauté mode until it thickens.
13. Serve the pork with this sauce on top.
14. Enjoy.

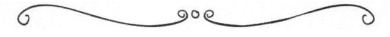

Burrito Beef
Prep + Cook time: 25 minutes | Serves: 4

Nutritional Info (per serving)

Calories	Fat (g)	Protein (g)	Carbs (g)
305	19.4	24.6	8.7

Ingredients:

2 pounds grass-fed, grass-finished ground beef

2 Tbs. olive oil

1 cup chopped onion

4 garlic cloves, minced

4 Tbs. chili powder

1 teaspoon ground cumin

2 teaspoon salt

1 teaspoon onion powder

1/2 teaspoon garlic powder

Directions:

1. Preheat the oil in a suitably sized cooking pot.
2. Add onion to sauté until golden.
3. Stir in garlic and sauté more for 1 min.
4. Add the beef along with all the spices.
5. Stir cook the mixture until the beef is al dente.
6. Enjoy.

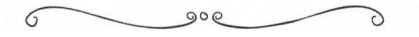

Mocha Spiced Pot Roast
Prep + Cook time: 45 minutes | Serves: 4

Nutritional Info (per serving)

Calories	Fat (g)	Protein (g)	Carbs (g)
420	25.1	25.7	24.7

Ingredients:

For the mocha rub:

2 tbs. finely ground coffee

2 tbs. smoked paprika

1 tbs. freshly ground black pepper

1 tbs. cocoa powder

1 teaspoon chili powder

1 teaspoon ground ginger

1 teaspoon of sea salt

For the roast:

2 pounds beef chuck roast, diced into 1½- to 2-inch cubes

1 cup brewed coffee

1 cup beef broth or bone broth

1 small onion, chopped

6 dried figs, chopped

3 tbs. balsamic vinegar

Kosher salt

Freshly ground black pepper

Directions:

1. Combine all the ingredients for the mocha rub in a bowl and set it aside.
2. Season the beef cubes with 4 tbs. of mocha rub and coat them well.
3. Blend the brewed coffee with figs, vinegar, onion, and broth in a blender.
4. Place the beef in the pressure cooker and pour the coffee sauce over it.
5. Secure the lid and select "Meat/ stew" function to cook.

6. Once done, release the pressure completely then remove the lid.
7. Roughly shred the meat using a fork.
8. Serve warm.

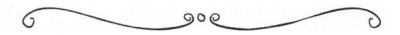

Pork Carnitas Bowl
Prep + Cook time: 45 minutes | Serves: 6

Nutritional Info (per serving)

Calories	Fat (g)	Protein (g)	Carbs (g)
449	15.3	71	2.6

Ingredients:

3 lbs. pork butt

1 Tbs. dried oregano

1 teaspoon Ceylon cinnamon

1/2 teaspoon ground cloves

2 dried bay leaves

1 1/2 teaspoon kosher salt

4 garlic cloves

1/2 yellow onion

1/2 cup water

Juice of one lemon

Juice of one lime

Directions:

1. Mix every spicein a bowl and set them aside.
2. Pat fry the pork using a paper towel and dice it into pieces.
3. Place the pork in the Instant along with mixed spices, citrus, onion, juices, garlic, and water.
4. Secure the lid and select Manual function for 30 minutes

5. Once done, release the pressure completely then remove the lid.
6. Serve warm.

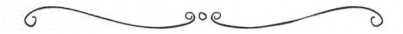

Ginger Pork Tenderloin
Prep + Cook time: 35 minutes | Serves: 2

Nutritional Info (per serving)

Calories	*Fat (g)*	*Protein (g)*	*Carbs (g)*
432	7.6	55.9	29.8

Ingredients:

½ cups Coconut Aminos

1 tbs. peel and dice Ginger, Fresh

2 tbs. Honey

2 tbs. Lemon Juice

½ cups chopped Cilantro, Fresh

2 teaspoons minced Garlic, Cloves

1 ½ pound quarter Pork Tenderloin

Directions:

1. Mix coconut aminos, ginger, honey, lemon juice, garlic and cilantro in a bowl.
2. Add pork to this marinade and mix well.
3. Marinate the pork for 2 hours in the refrigerator.
4. Place the pork in the baking pan and pour the marinade on top.
5. Bake the tenderloin for 20 minutes in the preheated oven.
6. Serve warm.

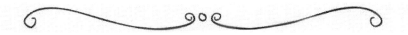

Herbed Pork Chops
Prep + Cook time: 25 minutes | Serves: 4

Nutritional Info (per serving)

Calories	Fat (g)	Protein (g)	Carbs (g)
245	13.9	21.5	8.8

Ingredients:

4 bone-in pork loin chops

1/2 teaspoon sea salt

1/4 teaspoon ground black pepper

1 tbs. fresh rosemary, diced

1 tbs. almond butter

2 tbs. extra virgin olive oil

1 large red onion, halved and sliced

1/2 cup balsamic vinegar

1 tbs. honey

Directions:

1. Let your oven preheat at 350 degrees F.
2. Season the pork chops with rosemary, pepper, and salt.
3. Heat butter with olive oil in a skillet and sear the chops for 4 minutes per side.
4. Transfer the chops to a plate then toss in onion.
5. Sauté for 1 minute then add honey and vinegar.
6. Stir cook until the sauce bubbles.
7. Return the cooked pork chops to the pan and transfer the pan to the oven.
8. Bake them for 15 minutes.
9. Serve warm.

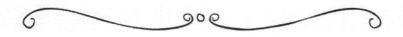

Roasted Pork Chops
Prep + Cook time: 35 minutes | Serves: 4

Nutritional Info (per serving)

Calories	*Fat (g)*	*Protein (g)*	*Carbs (g)*
345	23.3	34.4	1.1

Ingredients:

4 boneless pork chops 1 inch thick

4 tbs. extra virgin olive oil

2 teaspoons salt

1 teaspoon black pepper

1 teaspoon smoked paprika

1 teaspoon onion powder

Directions:

1. Let your oven preheat at 400 degrees F. grease the baking sheet with cooking spray.
2. Season the pork chop with spices and olive oil.
3. Place the chops in the baking sheet and bake them for 20 minutes.
4. Serve warm.

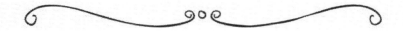

Crispy Dredged Pork Chops
Prep + Cook time: 25 minutes | Serves: 2

Nutritional Info (per serving)

Calories	Fat (g)	Protein (g)	Carbs (g)
355	22.6	26.1	12.5

Ingredients:

2 tbs. almond flour

1/4 teaspoon salt

1/4 teaspoon pepper

2 boneless pork loin chops

2 tbs. almond butter

1/4 teaspoon rubbed sage

1/8 teaspoon dried rosemary, crushed

1/2 cup sliced onion

1/2 cup unsweetened apple juice

2 tbs. chopped walnuts

Directions:

1. Mix 2 tbs. flours with salt, and peppers in a Ziplock bag.
2. Add pork chops and seal the bag. Shake the bag to coat the chops well.
3. Heat the almond butter in a skillet and sear the chops for 5 minutes per side.
4. Top them with rosemary and sage.
5. Transfer the chops to the serving plate.
6. Add onion to the same pan and sauté until soft.
7. Stir in remaining flour mixture, and juices. Stir cook until smooth.
8. Add nuts and cook for 2 minutes until it thickens.
9. Pour the sauce over the chops.
10. Serve warm.

Pork Chops and Apples

Prep + Cook time: 25 minutes | Serves: 4

Nutritional Info (per serving)

Calories	Fat (g)	Protein (g)	Carbs (g)
315	17.5	16.6	24.8

Ingredients:

4 1/2-inch-thick bone-in pork chops (4 ounces each)

2 teaspoons chopped fresh sage

salt and fresh ground pepper, to taste

2 tbs. extra-virgin olive oil, divided

2 apples, thinly sliced

1 large yellow onion, thinly sliced

1 teaspoon fresh rosemary, chopped

1/2 teaspoon fresh thyme, chopped

salt and fresh ground pepper, to taste

3/4 cup apple cider

Directions:

1. Liberally season the chops with salt, pepper,and sage from both the sides.
2. Preheat cooking oil in an iron skillet and sear the pork chops for 4 mins per side.
3. Transfer the cooked chops to any plate and keep them aside.
4. Add apples, remaining oil, and onions to the same pan.
5. Season this mixture with salt, pepper, thyme, and rosemary.
6. Stir cook the apples for 5 minutes then add cider.
7. Return the chops to the pan and cook for 5 minutes.

8. Serve warm.

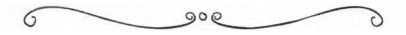

Beef Hamburger Soup
Prep + Cook time: 15 minutes | Serves: 6

Nutritional Info (per serving)

Calories	*Fat (g)*	*Protein (g)*	*Carbs (g)*
287	7.2	35.6	18

Ingredients

1 1/2 pounds minced beef

1 onion, chopped

3 sweet potatoes, peeled and diced

2 carrots, diced

2 stalks celery, chopped

1 bay leaf

1/4 teaspoon thyme

1/4 teaspoon dried basil

1 teaspoon salt

1/4 teaspoon pepper

6 cups water or broth

Directions:

1. Sauté ground beef in a greased until brown then transfer to the pressure cooker.
2. Add onion, potatoes, bay leaf, celery, carrots, and broth.
3. Secure the lid and pressure cook the beef for 4 minutes.
4. Release the pressure completely.
5. Add pepper, salt, basil, and thyme.
6. Enjoy.

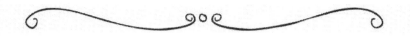

Pear Balsamic Pork

Prep + Cook time: 25 minutes | Serves: 4

Nutritional Info (per serving)

Calories	*Fat (g)*	*Protein (g)*	*Carbs (g)*
445	15.9	51.6	22.8

Ingredients:

4 tbs. avocado, divided

4 small pears, peeled, halved, and cored

2 (12-ounce) (grain-fed/grain finished) pork tenderloins, trimmed

1¼ teaspoons kosher salt

¼ teaspoon ground black pepper

⅛ teaspoon ground red pepper

⅓ cup Cinnamon Pear Balsamic Vinegar

1 tbs. finely chopped fresh sage

1 tbs. chopped fresh thyme leaves

Garnish: fresh sage and thyme sprigs

Directions:

1. Let your oven preheat at 375 degrees F.
2. Spray a 13x9 inch baking dish with cooking oil.
3. Heat 2 tbs. avocado oil in a large skillet, add the pears and cook it for 2 minutes.
4. Remove the pear from the skillet and place it in the plate.

5. Season the pork with pepper and salt, place the pork in the same pan.
6. Cook it for 4 minutes with occasional stirring.
7. Place the pear, pork in the baking dish and top it with vinegar, thyme, and sage.
8. Drizzle the remaining avocado oil.
9. Bake the pork for 18 minutes.
10. Garnish as desired.
11. Enjoy.

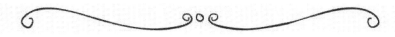

Cuban Pork Tacos
Prep + Cook time: 35 minutes | Serves: 2

Nutritional Info (per serving)

Calories	Fat (g)	Protein (g)	Carbs (g)
549	23.5	66.3	15.9

Ingredients:

For the Cuban Pork Marinade:

1/4 cup cilantro, chopped

2 tbs. olive or avocado oil

3 garlic cloves

1/2 teaspoon cumin

1/4 teaspoon dried oregano

1/2 teaspoon red pepper or cayenne

2–3 tbs. lime juice

1/2 cup orange juice

For pork

1 small white onion chopped

1 lb. lean pork or pork loin

avocado slices

dash of salt and black pepper 1/2teaspoon or less

1 cup shredded purple cabbage

Directions:

1. Blend all the ingredients for marinade in the blender.
2. Add pork, onion, pepper, salt, oil, and marinade in the pressure cooker.
3. Secure the lid and select Manual settings for 30 minutes at high pressure.
4. Once done, the release pressure naturally then remove the lid.
5. Garnish with your favorite toppings.

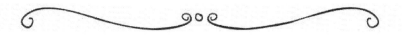

Pork Souvlaki Skewers

Prep + Cook time: 35 minutes | Serves: 4

Nutritional Info (per serving)

Calories	*Fat (g)*	*Protein (g)*	*Carbs (g)*
565	19.7	88.7	1.9

Ingredients:

2 1/2 pounds boneless pork sirloin chops

2 tbs. olive oil

Marinade:

1/2 cup olive oil

1/2 cup fresh lemon juice

1 tbs. red wine vinegar

1 tbs. dried oregano

1 tbs. garlic, minced

salt and ground black pepper to taste

Directions:

1. Dice the pork into cubes and place them in a Ziploc bag.
2. Add all the marinade ingredients and crushed oregano, seal the bag.
3. Shake well to coat the pork and marinate it for 6 hours in the refrigerator.
4. Drain the pork and thread it on the skewers.
5. Prepare and preheat the grill on medium heat.
6. Brush the skewers with olive then place them in the grill.
7. Cook the skewers for 15 minutes while rotating them every 5 minutes.
8. Serve warm with your favorite salad.

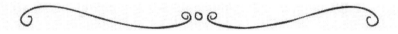

Pork Steaks with Mushrooms
Prep + Cook time: 25 minutes | Serves: 4

Nutritional Info (per serving)

Calories	Fat (g)	Protein (g)	Carbs (g)
416	31.7	26.5	8.4

Ingredients:

4 large, bone-in pork steaks (about 2 lbs.)

2 teaspoon lemon pepper seasoning

1 1/2 teaspoon sea salt, more to taste

3 tbs. almond butter

3 tbs. olive oil

1 cup chicken stock

6 cloves garlic, minced

8 oz. cremini mushrooms, quartered

2 tbs. fresh parsley, chopped

1 lemon, thinly sliced

Directions:

1. Season the pork steaks with lemon pepper seasoning and salt.
2. Heat fats in the cooking pan and sear the seasoned pork in it until brown from both the sides.
3. Transfer the cooked pork to any plate and add more fats to the pan.
4. Stir in ½ cup stock and deglaze the pan.
5. Add mushrooms and garlic, sauté for 3 minutes then add remaining stock.
6. Toss in lemon slices and cook the mixture for 5 minutes on a simmer.
7. Pour this sauce over the pork steaks.

Garlic Butter Pork Chops
Prep + Cook time: 25 minutes | Serves: 2

Nutritional Info (per serving)

Calories	Fat (g)	Protein (g)	Carbs (g)
324	27	18.3	1.9

Ingredients:

2 medium pork chops

kosher salt and freshly ground black pepper

4 tbs. grass-fed butter, melted

1 tbs. fresh thyme, chopped

2 cloves garlic, minced

1 tbs. olive oil, extra virgin

Directions:

1. Let your oven preheat oven to 375 degrees F.
2. Rub the pork chops with pepper and salt.
3. Mix thyme, butter, and garlic in a bowl.
4. Pour oil in an iron skillet and heat it.
5. Add the pork chops and sear it for 2 minutes per side.
6. Stir in a garlic mixture then transfer the pan to the oven.
7. Bake them for 12 minutes then serve.

Brussels Sprouts Lamb Stew
Prep + Cook time: 35 minutes | Serves: 4

Nutritional Info (per serving)

Calories	*Fat (g)*	*Protein (g)*	*Carbs (g)*
494	23.7	40.1	35

Ingredients:

4 tbs. extra virgin olive oil divided

1 onion diced

1 carrot diced

1 stalk celery diced

1-2 pounds lamb stew meat cut into one-inch cubes

1/4 cup almond flour

1 cup gluten-free chicken broth

1 8- ounce can tomato sauce

1 teaspoon parsley

1/2 teaspoon mint flakes

1/2 teaspoon dill weed

1/8 teaspoon cinnamon

1 teaspoon salt

dash of pepper

1 pound of brussels sprouts

Directions:

1. Sauté celery, onion, and carrots in 3 tbs. oil in a pan for 4 minutes.
2. Transfer this mixture to an Instant Pot.
3. Coat the lamb with flour and sear it in a greased pan until brown.
4. Transfer the lamb to the Instant Pot.
5. Pour in tomato sauce, broth and seasoning. Mix it all gently.
6. Secure the lid and select Manual mode for 20 minutes at high pressure.
7. Once done, release the pressure completely then remove the lid.
8. Add brussels sprouts to the mixture and mix well.
9. Serve warm.

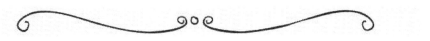

Bacon Braised Lamb Stew
Prep + Cook time: 60 minutes | Serves: 4

Nutritional Info (per serving)

Calories	Fat (g)	Protein (g)	Carbs (g)
888	25.1	85.5	72.8

Ingredients:

2 oz. uncured bacon strips

2 tbs. tapioca flour

1 1/2 lbs. of lamb or lamb loin, diced

1/2 teaspoon black pepper

1/2 sea salt (or to taste)

1 cup chopped onion

1/2 teaspoon garlic minced

3 1/2 cup chicken or vegetable stock

1 cup carrots, chopped

1 cup celery, chopped

1/4 teaspoon dried thyme

2 cups sweet potato, chopped

1 bay leaf

Directions:

1. Sauté the bacon strips in a stock pot until crispy.
2. Transfer the bacon to a plate and crumble it into pieces once cooled.
3. Remove half of the bacon fats from the pot and add lamb, dusted with flour.
4. Cook the lamb from both sides until brown and tender. It takes 10 minutes.
5. Add reserved bacon fat to the pot along with garlic, onion, pepper, and salt.
6. Stir cook until the onion turns golden.
7. Add bacon and cover the pot to cook for 35 minutes on a simmer.
8. Stir in bay leaves, celery, carrots, thyme, and sweet potatoes.
9. Again, cover the pot to cook more for 20 minutes.
10. Adjust seasoning with salt and pepper and discard the bay leaves.
11. Enjoy warm.

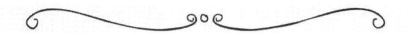

Lamb Vindaloo

Prep + Cook time: 25 minutes | Serves: 2

Nutritional Info (per serving)

Calories	Fat (g)	Protein (g)	Carbs (g)
441	26	22.2	29.1

Ingredients:

1 lb. lamb neck fillet, cubed

4 oz. rapeseed oil

2 onions, sliced

4 garlic cloves, roughly chopped

1-inch ginger, roughly chopped

For the curry paste

2 teaspoon cardamom pods shelled, seeds only

2 teaspoon cloves

2 teaspoon coriander seeds

1 medium sweet potato, diced

1 cup stock, warmed through

1 teaspoon coriander, chopped

1 teaspoon cumin seeds, toasted

1 teaspoon turmeric

1 tbs. malt vinegar

2 teaspoon dried red chilies

Directions:

1.   Blend all the ingredients for curry paste in a blender until smooth.

2. Rub this mixture over the lamb neck and cover it to marinate in the refrigerator overnight.

3. Preheat oil in a saucepan and sauté garlic, ginger, and onion until soft.

4. Stir in the remaining curry paste and stir cook for 1 minute.

5. Toss in sweet potatoes and sauté for 5 minutes.

6. Pour in stock and let it simmer on low heat until the potato is tender.

7. Sear the marinated lamb neck in a greased pan until al dente.

8. Reheat the vegetable curry and pour over the lamb.

9. Garnish with coriander and serve.

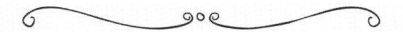

Moroccan Lamb Casserole

Prep + Cook time: 45 minutes | Serves: 4

Nutritional Info (per serving)

Calories	Fat (g)	Protein (g)	Carbs (g)
741	50.6	28.2	48.1

Ingredients:

1 tbs. coconut oil

1 medium white onion, chopped

1/2 teaspoon salt

1.5 lb. lamb steak, diced

4 peels of lemon

1 teaspoon cinnamon powder

1 1/2 teaspoon cumin powder

1 1/2 teaspoon coriander seed powder

1/2 teaspoon allspice

1 teaspoon onion powder

2 tbs. lemon juice

2 large cloves of garlic, sliced

6–7 dried apricots, sliced in thirds

1 tbs. tomato sauce

2 bay leaves

1 1/2 cups water

1 teaspoon salt

1/4 cup toasted almond slivers

A handful of chopped fresh parsley

Directions:

1. Sauté onion for 2 minutes in heated coconut oil pressure cooker.
2. Stir in all the spices, lamb, lemon peel and carrots. Sauté it for a minute.
3. Add water, tomato sauce, garlic and apricot to the lamb.
4. Secure the lid and cook on Manual mode for 25 minutes at high pressure.
5. Once done release the pressure completely then remove the lid.
6. Add the almond and parsley and mix well then serve warm.

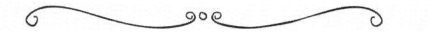

Coconut Lamb Curry
Prep + Cook time: 35 minutes | Serves: 4

Nutritional Info (per serving)

Calories	*Fat (g)*	*Protein (g)*	*Carbs (g)*
471	39.3	18.3	14.1

Ingredients:

1 tbs. coconut oil

1.5 lb. diced lamb boneless

1 large brown onion, diced

1/2 long red chili, finely diced

2 medium celery sticks, diced

3 cloves garlic, diced

2 1/2 teaspoons garam masala powder

1 1/4 teaspoons turmeric powder

1 teaspoon fennel seeds

1 1/2 teaspoons coconut oil

1 ½ cup of coconut milk

1 1/2 tbs. tomato sauce

1 cup of water

1 1/3 teaspoon sea salt

2 medium carrots, diced

A squeeze of lime or lemon juice

parsley to garnish

Directions:

1. Grease a pressure cooker with cooking oil and heat it on medium heat.
2. Place the lamb in the saucepan and cook it for 4 minutes until it is brown.
3. Stir in celery, chili,and onion, sauté for a minute.
4. Add fennel seeds, turmeric, garlic, garam masala, and coconut oil.
5. Stir in gently then add tomato sauce, carrot, salt, water, and coconut milk.
6. Secure the lid and select Manual mode for 25 minutes at high pressure.
7. Once done, release the pressure completely then remove the lid.
8. Add coriander and lemon juice.
9. Serve warm.

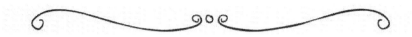

Irish Lamb Stew

Prep + Cook time: 55 minutes | Serves: 6

Nutritional Info (per serving)

Calories	*Fat (g)*	*Protein (g)*	*Carbs (g)*
523	19.3	59.8	24.1

Ingredients:

2 1/2 lb. lamb shoulder cubed

4 slices bacon sliced into 1-inch pieces

2 onions cut into wedges

2 lbs. sweet potatoes peeled and quartered

6 carrots peeled and sliced

1 turnip cubed

4 cups chicken beef or vegetable stock

1 teaspoon dried thyme

salt and pepper to taste

Directions:

1. Season the meat chunks with salt and pepper. Keep it aside.
2. Preheat a pressure cooker and sauté bacon for 4 minutes until crispy.
3. Transfer the crispy bacon to a plate lined with paper towel.
4. Add lamb to the pressure cooker and sear the chunks for 3 minutes until golden brown.
5. Remove the lamb and transfer it to a plate.
6. Add onion to the same cooker and sauté for 3 minutes.
7. Return the cooked lamb to the pot, along with thyme, turnip, carrots, potatoes, and broth.

8. After boiling the mixture, secure the lid.
9. Select the Manual mode to cook the lamb for 45 minutes on high pressure.
10. Release the pressure completely then remove the lid.
11. Serve warm.

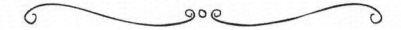

Seafood Recipes

Catfish with Tartar Sauce

Prep + Cook time: 25 minutes | Serves: 4

Nutritional Info (per serving)

Calories	*Fat (g)*	*Protein (g)*	*Carbs (g)*
381	21.9	34.4	8.7

Ingredients:

Cooking spray

4 (6-ounce) farm-raised catfish fillets

2 teaspoons Cajun seasoning

1/8 teaspoon salt

1/2 cup lectin free mayonnaise

1 tbs. sweet pickle relish

1 tbs. minced fresh onion

1 tbs. capers, drained

1/4 teaspoon dried oregano

Directions:

1. Heat a well-greased skillet on medium heat.
2. Season the fish with Cajun and salt seasoning liberally.
3. Place the seasoned fillets in the heated pan and cook for 4 minutes per side.
4. Transfer the cooked fish fillets to the serving plate.
5. Cook the fillets in batches to avoid the overcrowding of the pan.
6. Serve the fish with relish, onion, capers, and dried oregano mixed with mayonnaise.
7. Enjoy.

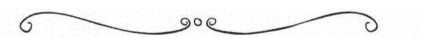

Tuna Niçoise Salad

Prep + Cook time: 25 minutes | Serves: 4

Nutritional Info (per serving)

Calories	*Fat (g)*	*Protein (g)*	*Carbs (g)*
699	14	44.6	104.5

Ingredients:

Salad:

4 ounces haricots green beans, trimmed

1 tbs. extra-virgin olive oil, divided

12 ounces sweet potato wedges

2 1/2 cups Bibb lettuce leaves

1/2 cup fresh basil leaves

1/2 cup red onion, thinly sliced

1/4 cup pitted kalamata olives, halved lengthwise

2 hard-cooked peeled eggs, quartered lengthwise (pasture raised)

2 (8-ounce) tuna steaks

1/8 teaspoon salt

1/8 teaspoon freshly ground black pepper

Dressing:

2 tbs. fresh lemon juice

1 tbs. water

1/2 teaspoon swerve

1/8 teaspoon salt

1/8 teaspoon freshly ground black pepper

1 garlic clove, minced

3 1/2 tbs. extra-virgin olive oil

1 tbs. capers

Directions:

1. Parboil green beans for 2 minutes in the boiling water then drain it instantly.
2. Take a large skillet with 1 teaspoon of cooking oil. stir in sweet potatoes.
3. Sauté for 5 minutes until golden brown.
4. Spread the lettuce leaves in the serving place then top them with green beans, eggs, olives, onion, and sweet potatoes.
5. Season tuna with salt and pepper. Sear it for 2 minutes per side in the heated greased pan.
6. Slice the seared tuna and place it on the lettuce salad.
7. Mix the remaining ingredients for dressing then pour it over the salad.
8. Enjoy.

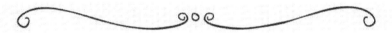

Salmon Fillets with Cauliflower
Prep + Cook time: 45 minutes | Serves: 6

Nutritional Info (per serving)

Calories	*Fat (g)*	*Protein (g)*	*Carbs (g)*
264	13.1	29.8	8.9

Ingredients:

6 cups cauliflower florets

2 tbs. olive oil

1/2 teaspoon freshly ground black pepper

1/4 teaspoon kosher salt, divided

3 tbs. Dijon mustard

1 tbs. honey

2 teaspoons chopped fresh dill

2 teaspoons fresh lemon juice

4 (6-ounce) sustainable salmon fillets

Cooking spray

Directions:

1. Let your oven preheat at 400 degrees F.
2. Toss cauliflower with salt and pepper in a baking sheet.
3. Bake them for 25 minutes in the heated oven while toasting after every 10 minutes.
4. Mix honey, mustard, juice, and dill in a suitably sized bowl.
5. Place the fish fillets in a baking pan lined with a foil sheet.
6. Drizzle salt and pepper on top to season the fish.
7. Pour the mustard mixture over the fillets.
8. Bake them for 17 minutes in the preheated oven.
9. Serve warm with cauliflower.

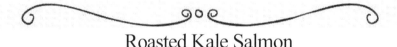

Roasted Kale Salmon

Prep + Cook time: 25 minutes | Serves: 4

Nutritional Info (per serving)

Calories	Fat (g)	Protein (g)	Carbs (g)
552	23.4	49.6	38.4

Ingredients:

12 ounces sweet potatoes, diced

1 teaspoon sherry vinegar

3/4 teaspoon kosher salt, divided

2 smoked bacon slices, thinly sliced crosswise

1/2 cup shallots, finely chopped

1 tbs. olive oil

5 cups kale leaves, chopped

1/2 cup chicken stock, divided

1 teaspoon fresh rosemary, finely chopped

1/2 teaspoon freshly ground black pepper,

4 (6-ounce) skin-on salmon fillets

1/4 cupcoconut milk

4 fresh flat-leaf parsley sprigs

Directions:

1. Let your oven preheat at 425 degrees F.
2. Boil sweet potatoes in a pot filled with water and cook for 20 minutes on a simmer.
3. Drain the potatoes and place roughly crush each potato.
4. Season the potato mash with salt and vinegar.
5. Take a large skillet and sauté bacon for 3 minutes until crispy.
6. Stir in shallots and sauté for 3 minutes, transfer the mix to a plate.
7. Add potatoes mixture, kales, rosemary and ¼ cup stock to the skillet.
8. Cover the skillet to cook the mixture for 2 minutes on low heat.
9. Add the remaining stock, bacon mixture, pepper, and salt. Mix gently and keep it aside.
10. Season the fillets with salt and pepper.
11. Heat oil to sear the fish for 3-4 minutes per side in a pan.

12. Serve over warm, sweet potatoes mixture and garnish with parsley.
13. Enjoy

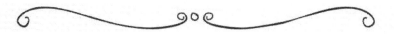

Halibut with Bacon Sauté
Prep + Cook time: 25 minutes | Serves: 4

Nutritional Info (per serving)

Calories	*Fat (g)*	*Protein (g)*	*Carbs (g)*
299	12.6	38.4	8.5

Ingredients:

1 tbs. extra-virgin olive oil

4 (6-ounce) skinless halibut fillets

1/4 teaspoon salt

1/4 teaspoon freshly ground black pepper

1 center-cut Applewood-smoked bacon slice

1 1/2 tbs. almond butter

3/4 cup (1-inch) sliced green onions

4 lime wedges

Directions:

1. Take a large skillet on medium heat and heat it with cooking oil.
2. Season the fish with black pepper and salt.
3. Sear the fish for 4 minutes per side in the skillet then transfer to plate.
4. Sauté bacon in the same pan for 4 minutes until crispy.
5. Add almond butter and cook for one minute.
6. Toss in green onions and sauté for 1 minute.

7. Serve the fish with sautéed bacon mixture and lime wedges.

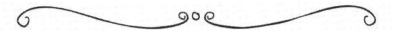

Grilled Shrimp with Vegetables
Prep + Cook time: 25 minutes | Serves: 4

Nutritional Info (per serving)

Calories	*Fat (g)*	*Protein (g)*	*Carbs (g)*
206	9.8	13.7	22.3

Ingredients:

3 tbs. almond milk

7 teaspoons extra-virgin olive oil, divided

3 tbs. minced fresh chives, divided

1 tbs. chopped fresh dill

1 teaspoon cider vinegar

1 teaspoon freshly ground black pepper, divided

3/4 teaspoon kosher salt, divided

1 teaspoon honey

16 large shrimp, peeled and deveined

20 large okra pods

Cooking spray

Directions:

1. Let your grill preheat at high heat.
2. Mix almond milk with 2 tbs. oil, chives, salt, pepper, dill and vinegar in a bowl.
3. Toss shrimp with honey and 1 teaspoon oil in a bowl.

4. Thread the seasoned shrimp on the skewers.
5. Similarly, thread the okra pods on the skewers.
6. Grill the okra skewers for 14 minutes while turning after every 4 minutes.
7. Grill the shrimp skewers for 3 minutes per side.
8. Pour chives mixture over the skewers.
9. Enjoy

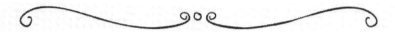

Shrimp and Kale Green Curry
Prep + Cook time: 25 minutes | Serves: 4

Nutritional Info (per serving)

Calories	*Fat (g)*	*Protein (g)*	*Carbs (g)*
499	34.1	16.9	33.8

Ingredients:

6 ounces dried rice noodles

2 teaspoons olive oil

1/3 cup chopped green onions

1 tbs. chopped fresh garlic

1 tbs. chopped fresh ginger

2 tbs. Thai green curry paste

1 1/4 cups carrots, julienned

1/2 cup unsalted chicken stock

1 (13.5-ounce) can light coconut milk

6 cups packed Lacinato kale, chopped

1/4 teaspoon kosher salt

1 pound peeled and deveined medium shrimp

1/4 cup chopped fresh cilantro

1 1/2 teaspoons fresh lime juice

1 teaspoon grated lime rind

Directions:

1. Cook the rice noodles as per the given instructions on the packet.
2. Rinse and drain the noodles and keep them aside.
3. Take a large skillet and preheat oil in it on medium heat.
4. Toss in green onion, ginger, garlic and sauté for 1 minute.
5. Stir in curry paste and stir cook for 30 seconds.
6. Add chicken stock, coconut milk, and carrots. Cook the mixture for 5 mins on a simmer.
7. Add salt and kale, cook more for 3 minutes.
8. Stir in shrimp and cook for another 3 minutes then add lime rind, juice, and cilantro.

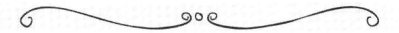

Flounder with Edamame and Bok Choy
Prep + Cook time:25 minutes | Serves: 4

Nutritional Info (per serving)

Calories	*Fat (g)*	*Protein (g)*	*Carbs (g)*
586	10	56.5	76.5

Ingredients:

2 teaspoons sesame oil

2 cups seafood stock

12 shiitake mushroom caps, thinly sliced

1 cup of water

2 tbs. mirin

1 1/2 tbs. white miso

2 teaspoons rice vinegar

3 garlic cloves, thinly sliced

1 (2-inch) piece ginger, thinly sliced

4 (6-ounce) flounder fillets

2 cups chopped baby bok choy

1 cup frozen shelled edamame, thawed

2 green onions, thinly diagonally sliced

2 teaspoons black or white sesame seeds

Directions:

1. Take a large saucepan and heat it with oil on medium heat.
2. Stir in mushrooms and sauté for 2 minutes.
3. Add stock and the next 6 ingredients.
4. Cook the mixture for 5 minutes on simmer.
5. Place the fish in the pan, bok choy and edamame.
6. Cover the vegetables with a lid and cook for 8 minutes on a simmer.
7. Garnish with green onions, and sesame seeds.
8. Enjoy.

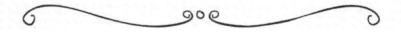

Indian Salmon
Prep + Cook time: 15 minutes | Serves: 4

Nutritional Info (per serving)

Calories	Fat (g)	Protein (g)	Carbs (g)
303	18.1	33.2	0.3

Ingredients:

1/2 teaspoon ground ginger

1/2 teaspoon garam masala

1/2 teaspoon ground coriander

1/4 teaspoon ground turmeric

Dash of kosher salt

Dash of ground red pepper

4 (6-ounce) skinless salmon fillets

Cooking spray

Directions:

1. Preheat your oven on broiler settings.
2. Combine all the ingredients in a small bowl except the fish fillets.
3. Rub the fillets with this mixture to season them well.
4. Then place them in a baking sheet greased with cooking oil.
5. Loosely cover the fillets with foil then broil for 7 minutes.
6. Serve warm.

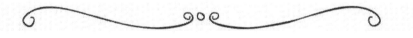

Basil Scallops
Prep + Cook time: 15 minutes | Serves: 2

Nutritional Info (per serving)

Calories	*Fat (g)*	*Protein (g)*	*Carbs (g)*
365	9.7	57.5	8.5

Ingredients:

1 cup chopped fresh basil

3/4 teaspoon kosher salt

1/4 teaspoon freshly ground
black pepper

1 tbs. canola oil

1 1/2 pounds sea scallops

Directions:

1. Take large cast iron and heat it on high heat with cooking oil.
2. Season the scallops with salt and pepper.
3. Sear the scallops in the pan for 2 minutes.
4. Garnish them with basil.
5. Enjoy.

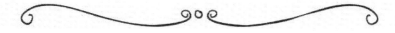

Smoked Plank Salmon
Prep + Cook time: 25 minutes | Serves: 4

Nutritional Info (per serving)

Calories	Fat (g)	Protein (g)	Carbs (g)
337	20.4	34.2	6.3

Ingredients:

1 (18-inch) cedar plank

1 small red onion, sliced

Cooking spray

3 tbs. chopped fresh cilantro

1/2 teaspoon kosher salt

1/2 teaspoon freshly ground black pepper

1 diced peeled avocado

1 lime, divided

4 (6-ounce) sustainable skinless salmon fillets

Directions:

1. Place the plank in water for 25 minutes then drain and set it aside.
2. Let your grill preheat on medium-high heat.
3. Grill the onion in the grill for 10 minutes.
4. Make sure to grease the grill and keep turning the veggies.
5. Remove the grilled vegetables and chop them.
6. Mix these vegetables with cilantro, salt, pepper, lime juice, and avocado.
7. Season the salmon with pepper and salt.
8. Place the plank in the grill for 3 minutes then flip it.
9. Place fish on its charred top and cover the grill to cook for 8 minutes.
10. Garnish the fish with grilled onion and lime wedges.
11. Enjoy.

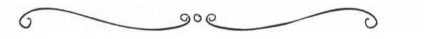

Sorghum Salmon

Prep + Cook time: 25 minutes | Serves: 4

Nutritional Info (per serving)

Calories	*Fat (g)*	*Protein (g)*	*Carbs (g)*
281	11	33.4	13

Ingredients:

3 tbs. sorghum

1 tbs. hot water

1 teaspoon dry mustard

1/4 teaspoon freshly ground black pepper

2 tbs. grated lemon zest

4 (6-ounce) salmon fillets

Cooking spray

3 tbs. fresh lemon juice (about 2 lemons)

1/2 teaspoon salt

Directions:

1. Let your oven preheat at 450 degrees F.
2. Mix sorghum with mustard, 1 tbs. hot water, lemon zest, salt and black pepper in a bowl.
3. Thoroughly coat both sides of the fillets with sorghum mixture.
4. Grease a baking pan and place the fillets in it.
5. Bake them for 9 minutes in the heated oven and baste them halfway through.
6. Switch the oven to broiler setting and broil the fillets for 1 minute.
7. Serve warm.

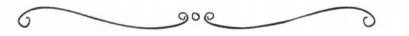

Scallops with Bacon and Spinach
Prep + Cook time: 15 minutes | Serves: 2

Nutritional Info (per serving)

Calories	Fat (g)	Protein (g)	Carbs (g)
501	14.3	70.9	25

Ingredients:

3 center-cut bacon slices

1 1/2 pounds jumbo sea scallops (about 12)

1/4 teaspoon kosher salt

1/4 teaspoon freshly ground black pepper

1 cup chopped onion

6 garlic cloves, sliced

12 ounces fresh baby spinach

4 lemon wedges (optional)

Directions:

1. Sauté bacon in a large cast iron skillet on medium heat until crispy.
2. Transfer the bacon to a plate and leave only 1 tbs. fats in the pan.
3. Chop the bacon and keep it aside.
4. Season the scallops with pepper and salt.
5. Sear these scallops in the pan for 2 minutes per side.
6. Transfer the scallops to a plate.
7. Toss the garlic and onion into the pan and sauté for 3 minutes.
8. Stir in spinach and cook it for 2 minutes.
9. Adjust seasoning with salt and pepper.
10. Divide the spinach in the serving plates.
11. Top this layer with scallops and bacon.
12. Serve warm.

Citrus Glazed Shrimp

Prep + Cook time: 15 minutes | Serves: 2-4

Nutritional Info (per serving)

Calories	*Fat (g)*	*Protein (g)*	*Carbs (g)*
321	11.7	43.5	16.1

Ingredients:

1-pound large shrimp, peeled and deveined

2 teaspoons minced garlic

2 teaspoons grated lime rind

1/4 teaspoon kosher salt

1/4 teaspoon chipotle chile powder

1/4 teaspoon freshly ground black pepper

Cooking spray

2 tbs. fresh lime juice

2 tbs. almond butter

Directions:

1. Toss shrimp with garlic, lime rind, salt, pepper, chili powder in a bowl.
2. Preheat a large greased pan and sauté shrimp for 3 minutes.
3. Add almond butter and lime juice. Cook for 1 minute.
4. Serve warm.

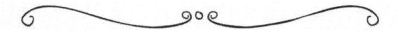

Tarragon Butter Sole
Prep + Cook time: 15 minutes | Serves: 4

Nutritional Info (per serving)

Calories	Fat (g)	Protein (g)	Carbs (g)
299	7.7	42.6	4.5

Ingredients:

4 (6-ounce) sole fillets

1/2 teaspoon salt, divided

1/4 teaspoon freshly ground black pepper

Cooking spray

3/4 cup dry white wine

3/4 cup fat-free, lower-sodium chicken broth

1/3 cup finely chopped shallots

1 tbs. minced fresh garlic

5 teaspoons almond butter, cut into small pieces

1 tbs. chopped fresh chives

1 1/2 teaspoons chopped fresh tarragon

Directions:

1. Season the fish with salt and pepper.
2. Preheat a large greased skillet and sear the fish for 2 minutes per side.
3. Keep the fish aside in a plate.
4. pour the wine into the same pan then add broth, shallots, and garlic.
5. Cook for 10 minutes then add butter, tarragon, and chives.
6. Pour this sauce over the fish and enjoy warm.

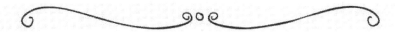

Black Grouper with Relish
Prep + Cook time: 15 minutes | Serves: 4

Nutritional Info (per serving)

Calories	Fat (g)	Protein (g)	Carbs (g)
338	14.6	39.5	11.6

Ingredients:

4 (6-ounce) black grouper fillets

1/2 teaspoon kosher salt, divided

1/4 teaspoon freshly ground black pepper

1 1/2 tbs. canola oil

1/3 cup thinly sliced radishes

2 tbs. chopped fresh chives

2 ripe peaches, peeled and cut into 1/2-inch chunks

1 serrano chile, thinly sliced

2 tbs. extra-virgin olive oil

1 tbs. fresh lime juice

2 teaspoons honey

Directions:

1. Preheat a large greased skillet on medium heat.
2. Season the fish liberally with salt and pepper.
3. Sear the fish for 2 minutes per side until golden in color.
4. Toss radishes with chives, and remaining ingredients.
5. Serve the fish with this relish on top.
6. Enjoy.

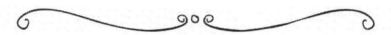

Shrimp Herb Salad

Prep + Cook time: 15 minutes | Serves: 2-4

Nutritional Info (per serving)

Calories	Fat (g)	Protein (g)	Carbs (g)
336	14.5	39.7	11.3

Ingredients:

Cooking spray

1-pound medium shrimp, peeled and deveined

3/8 teaspoon salt, divided

3 tbs. olive oil

2 tbs. fresh lemon juice

1/4 teaspoon freshly ground black pepper

1 (5-ounce) package mixed salad greens

1/4 cup basil leaves, chopped

2 tbs. coarsely chopped fresh oregano leaves

Directions:

1. Take a large greased skillet and cook shrimp for 2 minutes per side.
2. Mix oil with juice, salt, and pepper in a large enough bowl.
3. Toss in greens, oregano, and basil to the dressing.
4. Stir in the cooked shrimp and mix well gently.
5. Serve fresh.

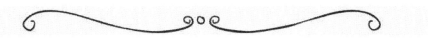

Salmon with Shallot Cream
Prep + Cook time: 15 minutes | Serves: 4

Nutritional Info (per serving)

Calories	Fat (g)	Protein (g)	Carbs (g)
512	27.2	66.6	1.7

Ingredients:

1/4 cup crème fraiche

2 tbs. finely minced shallots

1 tbs. almond milk

1 tbs. chopped fresh dill

1 1/2 teaspoons fresh lemon juice

1 1/8 teaspoons kosher salt, divided

1 (3-pound) boneless salmon fillet

1 tbs. olive oil

1/2 teaspoon freshly ground black pepper

1 tbs. chopped fresh chives

Directions:

1. Let your oven preheat at 450 degrees F.
2. Mix the first five ingredients along with 1/8 teaspoon salt in a suitably sized bowl.
3. Place the fish in the baking sheet lined with wax paper with its skin side down.
4. Rub the fish top with oil, salt, and pepper.
5. Bake them for 8 minutes in the preheated oven.
6. Switch the oven to broiler settings.
7. Broil the fish for 4 minutes.
8. Garnish it with shallot mixture and chives.
9. Serve warm.

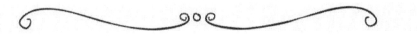

Orange Fennel Bass
Prep + Cook time: 45 minutes | Serves: 4

Nutritional Info (per serving)

Calories	Fat (g)	Protein (g)	Carbs (g)
402	12.9	61.2	7.7

Ingredients:

1 large fennel bulb with stalks

2 tbs. extra-virgin olive oil, divided

6 garlic cloves, minced

3/4 teaspoon kosher salt, divided

1/4 teaspoon freshly ground black pepper

2 (1 3/4-pound) whole cleaned striped bass

Cooking spray

1 orange, cut into 8 slices

3 tbs. fresh lemon juice

Directions:

1. Let your oven preheat at 400 degrees F.
2. Chop the fennel fronds and slice the fennel bulb.
3. Sauté sliced fennel in heated 1 tbs. oil in a pan.
4. Add garlic and sauté for 6 minutes then add salt. Allow this mixture to cool.
5. Score the fish skin with 3 cuts and
6. Brush the fish with lemon juice, salt, pepper, and oil, inside out.
7. Place the fish, fennel mixture and 4 orange slices in a greased baking pan.
8. Bake it for 30 minutes in the preheated oven.
9. Garnish with 1 tbs. fennel fronds.
10. Serve warm.

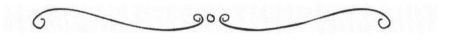

Shrimp Asparagus
Prep + Cook time: 15 minutes | Serves: 2

Nutritional Info (per serving)

Calories	*Fat (g)*	*Protein (g)*	*Carbs (g)*
254	8.5	31	13.3

Ingredients:

2 teaspoons olive oil

2 3/4 cups chopped sweet onion

2 garlic cloves, minced

1 3/4 cups (1/2-inch) slices asparagus

1 pound peeled and deveined medium shrimp, cut into 1-inch pieces

1/2 cup (2 ounces) crumbled feta cheese

1 tbs. chopped fresh dill

2 tbs. fresh lemon juice

1/8 teaspoon salt

1/8 teaspoon freshly ground black pepper

Directions:

1. Preheat a saucepan with oil in it on medium heat.
2. Toss in onion, sauté for 5 minutes then add garlic.
3. Toss in shrimp and asparagus. Cook it for 5 minutes.
4. Garnish with remaining ingredients.
5. Enjoy warm.

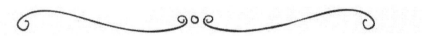

Grouper with Provençal Vegetables
Prep + Cook time: 25 minutes | Serves: 4

Nutritional Info (per serving)

Calories	*Fat (g)*	*Protein (g)*	*Carbs (g)*
241	4.8	42.9	4.4

Ingredients

2 cups fennel bulb, thinly sliced

2 tbs. fresh orange juice

16 picholine olives, pitted and chopped

1/2 teaspoon salt, divided

1/2 teaspoon black pepper, divided

Cooking spray

2 teaspoons olive oil

1 garlic clove, minced

4 (6-ounce) grouper fillets (about 1 inch thick)

Directions:

1. Let your oven preheat at 450 degrees F.
2. Combine salt, pepper, fennel bulb, orange juice, and olives in a bowl.
3. Spread this mixture in a baking pan and bake it for 5- 7 minutes.
4. Brush the fish with oil, garlic, salt, and pepper.
5. Place the seaoned fish in a baking pan and bake it for 10 minutes.
6. Serve warm with fennel mixture.
7. Enjoy.

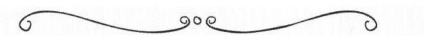

Crusted Cumin Sea Bass
Prep + Cook time: 25 minutes | Serves: 4

Nutritional Info (per serving)

Calories	Fat (g)	Protein (g)	Carbs (g)
357	8.7	63.5	3

Ingredients:

1 tbs. cumin seeds

1/2 teaspoon salt

1/4 teaspoon freshly ground black pepper

4 (6-ounce) white sea bass fillets

2 tbs. chopped fresh flat-leaf parsley

1/2 teaspoon olive oil

4 lemon wedges

Directions:

1. Let your oven preheat at 375 degrees F.
2. Toast cumin seeds in a large skillet for 2 minutes.
3. Transfer it to a grinder and grind well with salt and pepper.
4. Rub the fillets with this spice mixture.
5. Preheat a greased pan on medium temperature.
6. Place the fillets in the pan and cook for 2 minutes per side.
7. Cover the pan with aluminum foil and bake it for 4 minutes.
8. Garnish with lemon wedges and parsley.
9. Enjoy warm.

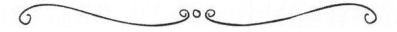

Shrimp with Lemony Greens
Prep + Cook time: 15 minutes | Serves: 2

Nutritional Info (per serving)

Calories	*Fat (g)*	*Protein (g)*	*Carbs (g)*
335	25.4	21.9	7.9

Ingredients:

1/2 cup olive oil

1 pinch red pepper

4 strips lemon zest

sea salt

2 cloves garlic sliced

1 pound wild-caught jumbo shrimp shells on

1/2 cup chopped fresh parsley

5 ounces mixed greens

white wine vinegar for sprinkling

Directions:

1. Combine oil, garlic, red pepper, lemon zest and salt in a pot.
2. Cook this mixture for 3 minutes until it sizzles.
3. Take another skillet and preheat it with little olive oil.
4. Sauté shrimp in it for 5 minutes until al dente.
5. Mix the lemon mixture with parsley and divide the mixture in the serving plates.
6. Top it with shrimps to serve.
7. Garnish with vinegar and white wine.
8. Enjoy.

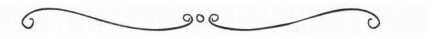

Tuna with Avocado Salad
Prep + Cook time: 25 minutes | Serves: 4

Nutritional Info (per serving)

Calories	*Fat (g)*	*Protein (g)*	*Carbs (g)*
652	46.7	49.5	10.4

Ingredients:

1/4 cup extra-virgin olive oil

zest and juice of 1/2 lemon

1/2 teaspoon honey

1 clove garlic, minced

1 small shallot, minced

1 teaspoon Italian seasoning

Himalayan sea salt and black pepper

4 wild-caught Yellowfin tuna steaks, 1/4 pound each

2 avocados, diced

2 cups loosely packed baby arugula

Directions:

1. Combine lemon juice, zest, honey, garlic, oil, shallots, salt, pepper shallot and Italian seasoning in a bowl.
2. Place the tuna steaks in a baking dish and brush them with half of the shallot's mixture.
3. Refrigerate them for 15 minutes.
4. Toss the arugula and avocados with the remaining shallots mixture.
5. Grill the tuna steaks for 4 minutes per side in a preheated grill.
6. Garnish with arugula and avocado.
7. Enjoy.

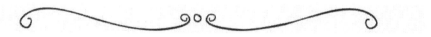

Shrimp Broccoli Stir Fry

Prep + Cook time: 25 minutes | Serves: 4

Nutritional Info (per serving)

Calories	*Fat (g)*	*Protein (g)*	*Carbs (g)*
283	7.4	40.4	12.2

Ingredients:

1/2 head cauliflower, riced

1 tbs. toasted sesame seeds

3 tbs. avocado oil

1 pound peeled and deveined wild-caught large shrimp

1 bunch scallions, sliced

1 teaspoon minced garlic

1 tbs. grated fresh ginger (2-inch piece)

1 bag broccoli (10 ounces), cut into 2-inch pieces

1/4 cup rice vinegar

1/4 cup unsalted vegetable broth

Directions:

1. Cook the cauliflower rice in the microwave in 5 minutes then add sesame seeds.
2. Preheat 1 tbs. oil in a suitably sized skillet on medium heat.
3. Toss in shrimp and sauté for 4 minutes.
4. Transfer the shrimp to a plate and keep them aside.
5. Heat up the remaining oil in the same pan and toss in scallions, broccoli, and ginger.
6. Sauté for 10 minutes then add broth and vinegar.
7. Cook for 2 minutes then add shrimp.
8. Stir cook for 1 minute.
9. Serve shrimp with cauliflower rice.
10. Enjoy.

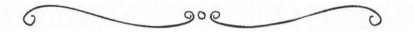

Blackened Shrimp
Prep + Cook time: 15 minutes | Serves: 1

Nutritional Info (per serving)

Calories	Fat (g)	Protein (g)	Carbs (g)
559	21.9	67.4	22

Ingredients:

1/2 lb. shrimp

½ tbs. blackening spice

1 tbs. avocado oil

1 tbs. almond butter

2 cloves minced garlic

1 cup almond milk

1/3 -1/2 cup grated parmesan cheese

2 cups arugula, to serve on the side

salt, to taste

Directions:

1. Wash, rinse and drain the shrimp. Season them with blackening spice.
2. Preheat a cast iron pan on medium-high heat with 1 tbs. avocado oil.
3. Toss in the seasoned shrimp and cook them for 4 minutes.
4. Sauté garlic with almond butter in another pan.
5. Pour in milk and parmesan. Cook until this sauce thickens.
6. Adjust seasoning with salt if needed.
7. Stir in cooked noodles and mix them well.
8. Serve the cooked shrimp with arugula.
9. Enjoy.

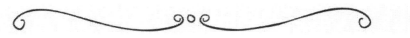

Shrimp Stuffed Avocado
Prep + Cook time: 5 minutes | Serves: 4

Nutritional Info (per serving)

Calories	Fat (g)	Protein (g)	Carbs (g)
275	20.4	14.3	12.3

Ingredients:

8 oz. salad shrimp

2 avocados

1 lime

2 tbs. lectin free mayo

1/2 teaspoon cumin

1/8 teaspoon oregano

2 tbs. finely chopped red onion

2 tbs. finely chopped celery

2 tbs. finely chopped red cabbage

salt & pepper, to taste

dash hot sauce, optional

2 teaspoon chopped cilantro

Directions:

1. Combine cumin, oregano, mayo, celery, onion, cabbage, salt, pepper, and lime juice.
2. Stir in hot sauce and mix it well.
3. Slice the avocados in half, remove the pit and stuff them with shrimp salad.
4. Top each half with onion mixture.
5. Serve fresh.

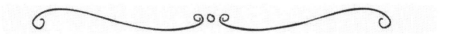

Blackened Shrimp Fajitas
Prep + Cook time: 15 minutes | Serves: 6

Nutritional Info (per serving)

Calories	Fat (g)	Protein (g)	Carbs (g)
347	16.5	37	13.9

Ingredients:

2 tbs. paprika

2 tbs. ancho chile powder

1 teaspoon dry mustard powder

1 teaspoon cayenne powder

4 teaspoons cumin

2 teaspoons black pepper

2 teaspoons dried oregano

1 teaspoon salt

1 teaspoon onion powder

1 teaspoon garlic powder

2 pounds shrimp

1 cup carrots, shredded

1 cup onions, sliced

2 avocados, diced

2 tbs. avocado oil

6 gluten-free flour tortillas

Directions:

1. Mix all the spices and shrimp in a bowl then let it sit for 5 minutes.
2. Sauté this mixture in a greased pan for 8 minutes.
3. Serve warm with onions, avocado and carrots in warm tortillas.
4. Enjoy.

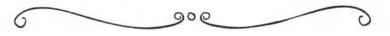

Grilled Alaska Coho Salmon
Prep + Cook time: 15 minutes | Serves: 4

Nutritional Info (per serving)

Calories	Fat (g)	Protein (g)	Carbs (g)
456	19.3	65	2.4

Ingredients:

2 pounds Alaska Coho salmon, (De-boned)

1 tbs. fresh thyme

2 teaspoons fresh chives

1 lime, (thinly sliced)

1/4 teaspoon Himalayan pink salt

2 teaspoons avocado oil

Directions:

1. Let your grill preheat at medium heat.
2. Place the salmon fillets on an aluminum sheet.
3. Top the fillets with lime slices, herbs, and salt.
4. Drizzle the oil on top and wrap the fish in its foil.
5. Place the fish in the grill for 8 minutes.
6. Serve warm.

Pesto Halibut Steak
Prep + Cook time: 15 minutes | Serves: 2

Nutritional Info (per serving)

Calories	Fat (g)	Protein (g)	Carbs (g)
443	16.9	68.5	2.3

Ingredients

2 halibut steaks, (Alaska)

1/2 teaspoon olive oil

3/4 cup fresh basil leaves

1 clove garlic

1 1/2 tbs. olive oil

1 1/2 tbs. toasted pine nuts

1 1/2 tbs. parmesan cheese

Salt to taste

dash black pepper

Directions:

1. Let your grill preheat at medium temperature.
2. Spread a piece of foil sheet and place halibut steaks on it.
3. Brush the fish with oil and season it with salt and pepper.
4. Blend basil, garlic, parmesan cheese, 3 tbs. oil and pine nuts in a blender.
5. Spread this pesto over the fish.
6. Transfer the fish to the grill with the foil sheet.
7. Cover the lid to smoke it for 10 minutes.
8. Enjoy.

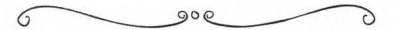

Vegetarian Recipes

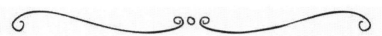

Turmeric Cauliflower Rice

Prep + Cook time: 15 minutes | Serves: 2

Nutritional Info (per serving)

Calories	Fat (g)	Protein (g)	Carbs (g)	Fiber (g)
248	5.7	1.5	14.4	0.2

Ingredients:

2 cups organic cauliflower rice

1 cup organic baby spinach (chopped)

1 tbs. organic red onion (diced)

2 cloves organic garlic (freshly crushed)

1 teaspoon organic ground black pepper

1/4 teaspoon organic ground turmeric

1/4 teaspoon Himalayan pink salt

Directions:

8. Toss everything into a wok along with cauliflower rice.
9. Adjust seasonings with salt and pepper.
10. Stir cook the mixture for 5 to 10 minutes until the rice is done.
11. Serve warm.

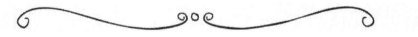

Roasted Cauliflower Steaks

Prep + Cook time: 65 minutes | Serves: 2

Nutritional Info (per serving)

Calories	Fat (g)	Protein (g)	Carbs (g)	Fiber (g)
249	11.8	6.9	12.8	1.1

Ingredients:

For the cauliflower

1 large head organic cauliflower, sliced

1 tbs. avocado oil

For the seasoning

1 tbs. organic dried dill

1/2 teaspoon organic ground cumin

1/4 teaspoon organic ground garlic powder

1/4 teaspoon organic ground black pepper

1/4 teaspoon Himalayan pink salt

For the tahini sauce

2 tbs. organic lemon juice

2 tbs. organic tahini

1/4 teaspoon organic dried dill

1/4 teaspoon organic ground black pepper

1/8 teaspoon Himalayan pink salt

Directions:

1. Let your oven preheat at 350 degrees F.
2. Spread the cauliflower chunks in a baking pan lined with wax paper.
3. Drizzle avocado oil over the cauliflower.

4. Mix all the seasonings together then drizzle it over the cauliflower.
5. Toss the cauliflower chunks well to coat them well.
6. Transfer the cauliflower to the oven for 60 minutes until golden brown.
7. Meanwhile, add all the tahini ingredients to a food processor.
8. Pour the tahini sauce over the cauliflower pieces.
9. Serve warm.

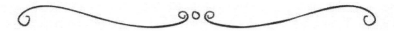

Pesto Sweet Potato

Prep + Cook time: 45 minutes | Serves: 2

Nutritional Info (per serving)

Calories	*Fat (g)*	*Protein (g)*	*Carbs (g)*	*Fiber (g)*
301	12.2	12.2	15	0.7

Ingredients:

For the sweet potatoes:

2 cups organic sweet potatoes, cubed

1pinch Himalayan pink salt

1pinch organic ground black pepper

For the cilantro pesto:

2 cups organic fresh cilantro

1/2 cup organic pine nuts

1/2 cup organic extra-virgin olive oil

1/3 cup nutritional yeast

3 cloves organic garlic

3 tbs. organic apple cider vinegar

1/2 teaspoon organic ground black pepper

1/2 teaspoon Himalayan pink salt

Directions:

1. Let your oven preheat at 350 degrees F.
2. Spread the potato cubes in a baking pan lined with parchment paper.
3. Drizzle salt and pepper over the potatoes.
4. Bake them for 35 minutes in the preheated oven.
5. Meanwhile, prepare the cilantro pesto.
6. Blend all the ingredients for pesto in a blender.
7. Drizzle pesto over baked potatoes.
8. Serve warm.

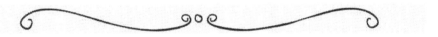

Cheesy Baked Mushrooms
Prep + Cook time: 25 minutes | Serves: 2

Nutritional Info (per serving)

Calories	Fat (g)	Protein (g)	Carbs (g)	Fiber (g)
276	18.5	13.1	12.5	0.7

Ingredients:

For the seasoning:

1/2 cup almond flour

1/2 cup nutritional yeast

1/4 - 1/2 teaspoon cayenne pepper, ground

1/2 teaspoon organic garlic powder, ground

1/2 teaspoon Himalayan
pink salt

Other:

2 cups organic baby Bella mushrooms (de-stemmed, sliced)

1 cup homemade almond milk

Directions:

1. Let your oven preheat at 425 degrees F.
2. Mix everything for the seasoning in a suitable bowl.
3. Slice the mushrooms and place them in a bowl.
4. Add almond milk to one bowl and keep half of the seasonings ready aside.
5. Dip mushrooms in the milk then coat them with seasoning mixture.
6. Once coated well, place the mushrooms in a baking sheet lined with wax paper.
7. Bake the coated mushrooms for 10 minutes in the preheated oven.
8. Flip the mushrooms then bake them again for 10 minutes.
9. Serve warm.

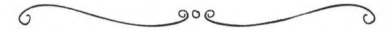

Basil and Artichoke Pasta
Prep + Cook time: 15 minutes | Serves: 2

Nutritional Info (per serving)

Calories	*Fat (g)*	*Protein (g)*	*Carbs (g)*	*Fiber (g)*
373	11.1	10.4	7.9	0.2

Ingredients:

2 packs Shirataki Fettuccine Pasta (Miracle Noodles)

For the sauce:

1 1/4 cups organic pine nuts

3/4 cup homemade almond milk

2 tbs. organic lemon juice

2 tbs. nutritional yeast

2 cloves organic garlic (freshly crushed)

1 tbs. organic extra-virgin olive oil

1/2 teaspoon Himalayan pink salt

1/2 teaspoon organic ground black pepper

8 leaves fresh organic basil (chopped)

1 can artichoke hearts (chopped), (14-ounce can)

Directions:

1. Prepare and cook the miracle noodles as per the given instructions on the pack.
2. Add the sauce ingredients to a blender until it is smooth and creamy.
3. Drain the pasta and toss it into a bowl.
4. Pour in the sauce along with basil and artichoke.
5. Toss everything well.
6. Serve fresh.

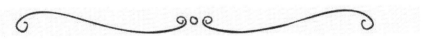

Cheesy Broccoli Bites
Prep + Cook time: 35 minutes | Serves: 3

Nutritional Info (per serving)

Calories	Fat (g)	Protein (g)	Carbs (g)	Fiber (g)
135	3.5	8.1	3.6	0.4

Ingredients

Broccoli:

3 cups broccoli florets

2 tbs. avocado oil

Seasoning:

1/4 cup almond flour

1/4 cup nutritional yeast

1/4 teaspoon organic ground garlic powder

1/8 teaspoon organic ground cayenne pepper

1/4 teaspoon Himalayan pink salt

Directions:

1. Let your oven preheat at 400 degrees F.
2. Combine all the ingredients for seasoning a bowl and set it aside.
3. Toss the broccoli floret with avocado oil and half of the seasoning mixture in a baking sheet.
4. Bake the florets for 10 minutes.
5. Add the remaining seasoning to the florets and toss them well.
6. Bake again for 25 minutes until crispy.
7. Serve warm.

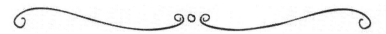

Cilantro Lime Cauliflower Rice
Prep + Cook time: 15 minutes | Serves: 2

Nutritional Info (per serving)

Calories	*Fat (g)*	*Protein (g)*	*Carbs (g)*	*Fiber (g)*
113	7.5	6.1	21.4	0

Ingredients:

2 cups organic cauliflower rice

2 tbs. organic lime juice

1 tbs. avocado oil

1 teaspoon Himalayan pink salt

1/2 teaspoon organic ground black pepper

1/4 cup organic fresh cilantro (chopped)

Directions:

1. Add everything to a wok or skillet except cilantro.
2. Stir cook this mixture for 5 minutes until it is done.
3. Garnish with cilantro.
4. Serve warm.

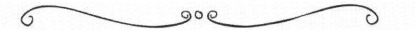

Shirataki Pasta with Avocado Sauce
Prep + Cook time: 15 minutes | Serves: 4

Nutritional Info (per serving)

Calories	*Fat (g)*	*Protein (g)*	*Carbs (g)*	*Fiber (g)*
276	6	2.7	26.1	0.6

Ingredients:

2 packs Shirataki (Miracle Noodles) Angel Hair Pasta

For the sauce:

2 organic avocados

1/4 cup organic extra-virgin olive oil

2 tbs. organic lime juice

1/2 - 1 teaspoon organic ground chipotle powder

1/4 teaspoon sea salt

Directions:

1. Prepare and cook the pasta as per the packet's direction.
2. Blend all the ingredients for sauce in a blender until smooth.
3. Drain the pasta and toss it into the medium bowl.
4. Add the prepared sauce to the pasta.
5. Stir it well then add cilantro or spinach.
6. Serve.

Mushroom Cauliflower Risotto
Prep + Cook time: 15 minutes | Serves: 2

Nutritional Info (per serving)

Calories	Fat (g)	Protein (g)	Carbs (g)	Fiber (g)
233	3.7	5.4	10.6	1.6

Ingredients:

1 1/2 cups organic baby Bella mushrooms (diced)

1/2 cup organic red onion (diced)

2 cloves organic garlic (freshly crushed)

2 tbs. organic extra-virgin olive oil

1 teaspoon Himalayan pink salt

1 teaspoon organic ground black pepper

1/2 teaspoon organic ground sage

1 can organic full-fat coconut milk (13.5-ounce can)

4 cups organic cauliflower rice

Directions:

1. Take a large skillet and add everything except the coconut milk and cauliflower rice.
2. Sauté until the onions are soft.
3. Pour the coconut milk and cauliflower to the pan.
4. Stir cook the mixture until the cauliflower is al dente.
5. Adjust seasoning with salt and pepper.
6. Serve warm.

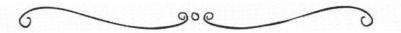

Pumpkin Spice Cauliflower Soup

Prep + Cook time: 25 minutes | Serves: 4

Nutritional Info (per serving)

Calories	*Fat (g)*	*Protein (g)*	*Carbs (g)*	*Fiber (g)*
289	3.1	6.8	16	0.3

Ingredients:

4 cups organic cauliflower rice

1/2 cup organic red onion (diced)

1 clove organic garlic (freshly crushed)

2 tbs. organic extra-virgin olive oil

2 teaspoons organic pumpkin spice

1 teaspoon organic dried rosemary

1/2 - 1 teaspoon Himalayan pink salt

1/2 teaspoon organic ground black pepper

1 can organic full-fat coconut milk (13.5-ounce can)

Directions:

1. Saute onions with garlic in olive oil in a heated pan.
2. Add rosemary, pepper, and salt and stir cook for 3 minutes.
3. Stir in cauliflower rice along with coconut milk and pumpkin spice.
4. Cook this mixture on a low simmer until the rice is al dente.
5. Adjust seasoning with salt, pepper, and rosemary.
6. Serve warm.

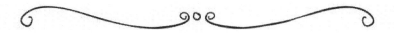

Artichoke Salad with Sesame Vinaigrette
Prep + Cook time: 35 minutes | Serves: 2

Nutritional Info (per serving)

Calories	Fat (g)	Protein (g)	Carbs (g)	Fiber (g)
178	11.5	13.1	10.4	0.1

Ingredients:

For the artichokes:

1 can artichoke hearts (14 ouncescandrain)

1 tbs. avocado oil

For the seasoning:

1/8 teaspoon Himalayan pink salt

1/8 teaspoon black pepperground

1/8 teaspoon garlic powderground

1/8 teaspoon paprikaground

For the vinaigrette:

1 tbs. organic sesame seeds

2 tbs. 100% pure avocado oil

2 tbs. organic apple cider vinegar

1 organic shallot (diced)

1 tbs. organic erythritol syrup

1/8 teaspoon Himalayan pink salt

1/8 teaspoon organic black ground pepper

For the salad:

2 cups organic mixed salad greens

Directions:

1. Let your oven preheat at 425 degrees F.

2. Thoroughly mix salt, pepper, paprika and garlic powder in a suitable bowl.
3. Drain the artichokes and cut them into quarter pieces.
4. Toss the artichokes with avocado oil and the prepared seasoning.
5. Spread the artichokes in a baking pan lined with parchment paper.
6. Bake them for 30 minutes 425 degrees F.
7. Toss the artichoke once it is baked halfway through.
8. Return the baking pan to the oven.
9. Meanwhile, mix all the vinaigrette ingredients in a suitable bowl.
10. Transfer the baked artichokes to the serving bowls.
11. Pour in the prepared vinaigrette.
12. Toss in the salad greens.
13. Mix it gently then serve fresh.

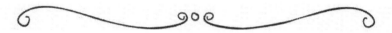

Sweet Potato with Spicy Guacamole
Prep + Cook time: 35 minutes | Serves: 2

Nutritional Info (per serving)

Calories	Fat (g)	Protein (g)	Carbs (g)	Fiber (g)
126	9.3	5.4	6.1	0.3

Ingredients:

For the sweet potato:

1 large organic sweet potato

1 - 2 teaspoons 100% pure avocado oil

For the guacamole:

2 organic avocados

1 tbs. organic red onion (diced)

1 tbs. organic cilantro (chopped)

2 cloves organic garlic (freshly crushed)

1/2 - 1 organic jalapeno (diced)

1 teaspoon organic lime juice (freshly squeezed)

1-2 pinches organic black ground pepper

1/4 teaspoon Himalayan pink salt

Directions:

1. Let your oven preheat at 350 degrees F.
2. Slice the sweet potatoes into ¼ inch thick slices.
3. Place these slices on a baking sheet and brush them with avocado oil.
4. Bake them for 30 mins in the preheated oven.
5. Flip the slices then bake again for 15 minutes.
6. Prepare the guacamole by mixing all of its ingredients.
7. Adjust seasonings as desired.
8. Place the baked potatoes in the serving dish and top it with guacamole.
9. Garnish with cilantro.
10. Serve fresh.

Creamy Mushroom Soup
Prep + Cook time: 25 minutes | Serves: 1

Nutritional Info (per serving)

Calories	Fat (g)	Protein (g)	Carbs (g)	Fiber (g)
273	12.1	1.6	15	0.2

Ingredients:

1 cup organic shitake mushrooms (sliced or diced)

1 cup organic baby Bella mushrooms (sliced or diced)

1/2 cup organic red onions (diced)

1 cup organic vegetable broth

1 can organic full-fat coconut milk (13.5-ounce can)

1 organic garlic clove (freshly crushed)

1 tbs. organic coconut aminos

2 teaspoons 100% pure avocado oil

1/2 teaspoon Himalayan pink salt

1/2 teaspoon organic ground black pepper

1/2 teaspoon organic dried thyme

Directions:

1. Take a medium sized pan and toss mushrooms with onions, garlic and avocado oil in it.
2. Add thyme, black and salt for seasoning. Mix them well.
3. Sauté the mushrooms for 3 minutes until soft.
4. Add coconut milk, coconut aminos, and vegetable broth to the mushrooms.
5. Cook them for 15 minutes on a medium simmer.
6. Adjust the seasoning with salt and pepper.
7. Garnish them pepper, green onions, and mushroom slices.
8. Serve fresh.

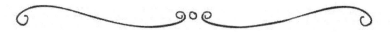

Sweet Potato Salad with Tahini Dressing
Prep + Cook time: 45 minutes | Serves: 4

Nutritional Info (per serving)

Calories	*Fat (g)*	*Protein (g)*	*Carbs (g)*	*Fiber (g)*
106	8.5	5.2	12.9	1.1

Ingredients:

1/2 organic avocado (sliced or cubed)

1 tbs. organic red onions (diced)

2 handfuls organic spring salad mix

For the sweet potatoes:

1 tbs. 100% pure avocado oil

1 teaspoon chipotle powder, ground

1/2 teaspoon organic ground garlic powder

1/4 teaspoon Himalayan pink salt

2 cups organic sweet potato,cubed

Dressing:

1/4 cup organic tahini

3 tbs. organic lime juice

2 tbs. filtered/purified water

1/4 teaspoon organic ground garlic powder

1/4 teaspoon Himalayan pink salt

1 - 2 pinches organic ground black pepper

Directions:

1. Let your oven preheat at 350 degrees F.
2. Peel and dice the sweet potatoes and keep them aside.
3. Toss the sweet potatoes with avocado oil, chipotle powder, salt, and garlic powder.
4. Mix them well to coat then spread them in a baking sheet.
5. Bake them for 25 minutes in the preheated oven.
6. Blend the tahini ingredients until it is smooth.
7. Dice the onion and avocado into cubes.
8. Serve the baked sweet potatoes with tahini, onion, and avocado on top.

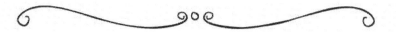

Spicy Lemon Broccolini
Prep + Cook time: 15 minutes | Serves: 2

Nutritional Info (per serving)

Calories	Fat (g)	Protein (g)	Carbs (g)	Fiber (g)
293	1.6	8.7	12.1	0.5

Ingredients:

2 cups organic broccolini

2 tbs. organic lemon juice (squeezed)

2 cloves organic garlic (freshly crushed)

1 teaspoon organic extra virgin olive oil

1/4 teaspoon Himalayan pink salt

1 pinch red pepper powder

Directions:

1. Prepare the broccolini by slicing off the stems.
2. Add everything to the skillet along with the broccolini.
3. Sauté them for 3 minutes.
4. Garnish with sesame seeds.
5. Enjoy.

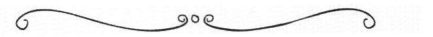

Chipotle Cauliflower Bake
Prep + Cook time: 65 minutes | Serves: 2

Nutritional Info (per serving)

Calories	Fat (g)	Protein (g)	Carbs (g)	Fiber (g)
178	3.1	4.7	10.4	1.1

Ingredients:

1 organic cauliflower

2 tbs. 100% pure avocado oil

1 organic lime

For the seasoning:

1/2-1 tbs. organic ground chipotle powder

1/4-1/2 teaspoon organic garlic powder

1/4-1/2 teaspoon Himalayan pink salt

Directions:

1. Let your oven preheat at 325 degrees F.
2. Combine all the ingredients for seasoning in a bowl and keep it aside.
3. Dice the cauliflower into bite-sized chunk and place them in a medium-sized bowl.
4. Toss the cauliflower with avocado oil and spread them in the baking sheet.

5. Sprinkle the veggies with seasonings.
6. Bake them for 60 minutes or more until soft.
7. Drizzle lemon juices on top.
8. Serve warm.

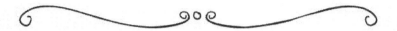

Almond Stuffed Brussels Sprouts
Prep + Cook time: 25 minutes | Serves: 4

Nutritional Info (per serving)

Calories	*Fat (g)*	*Protein (g)*	*Carbs (g)*	*Fiber (g)*
276	11.2	4.1	14.2	0.3

Ingredients:

15 - 20 organic brussels sprouts

Stuffing:

1 cup of organic almonds

1/4 cup olive oil

2 cloves organic garlic

2 tbs. organic lemon juice

2 tbs. nutritional yeast

1 tbs. organic apple cider vinegar

1 teaspoon organic ground chipotle

1/2 teaspoon Himalayan pink salt

Directions:

1. Slice the brussels sprouts into half and keep them aside.
2. Place the sprouts in some boiling water for 2 minutes then drain immediately.
3. Once cooled, remove the inner portion of each sprout half and keep the shell.

4. Grind the remaining ingredients in a food processor until crumbly.
5. Stuff the Brussels shells with this mixture.
6. Bake them for 20 mins at 400 degrees F in the preheated oven.
7. Serve warm.

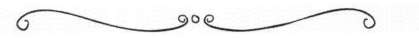

Avocado Mushroom Soup

Prep + Cook time: 25 minutes | Serves: 3

Nutritional Info (per serving)

Calories	*Fat (g)*	*Protein (g)*	*Carbs (g)*	*Fiber (g)*
356	0.9	3.5	8.1	0.3

Ingredients:

3 cups of water

3 cups of organic mushrooms

1 cup organic pine nuts

1 organic avocado (pitted)

1/2 cup organic red onion

2 cloves organic garlic

1 teaspoon organic fresh thyme

1 teaspoon Himalayan pink salt

1 teaspoon organic ground black pepper

Directions:

1. Blend everything in a food processor or a blender until smooth.
2. Transfer the pureed mixture to a stockpot.
3. Cook the soup for 15 minutes until it is partially cooked.

4. Garnish with chopped onions, pepper, and sliced mushrooms.
5. Serve warm.

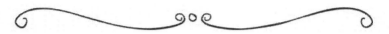

Spring Vegetable Alfredo
Prep + Cook time: 25 minutes | Serves: 4

Nutritional Info (per serving)

Calories	Fat (g)	Protein (g)	Carbs (g)	Fiber (g)
252	1.6	3.5	16.4	0

Ingredients:

4 servings of grain-free pasta

sea salt and black pepper, to taste

1/4 cup olive oil,

5 ounces shiitake mushrooms, cut in slices

1 bunch thin asparagus, trimmed and cut into 2-inch pieces

1 cup imported Italian mascarpone

1/4 cup grated Parmigiano-Reggiano

1/2 cup chopped fresh Italian parsley or basil leaves

1/2 teaspoon Italian seasoning

zest of 1/2 lemon

Directions:

1. Cook the pasta as per the given instruction on the packet.
2. Drain the pasta and reserve about 1 cup of cooking liquid.
3. Toss the pasta with cooking oil.
4. Preheat about 2 tbsp of olive oil in a skillet.

5. Toss in mushrooms and sauté them for 2 minutes.
6. Then stir in asparagus, salt, and olive oil.
7. Sauté for another 3 minutes.
8. Add noodles and mascarpone to the mushrooms.
9. Stir them then season the pasta with herbs, pecorino. Lemon zest and Italian seasoning.
10. Drizzle salt and pepper on top.
11. Serve fresh.

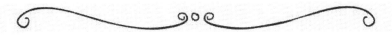

Shallot Caper Salad
Prep + Cook time: 5 minutes | Serves: 2

Nutritional Info (per serving)

Calories	Fat (g)	Protein (g)	Carbs (g)	Fiber (g)
155	13.3	6.7	3.8	0.4

Ingredients:

1 small shallot, finely chopped

2 tbs. capers, sliced

1 teaspoon minced garlic (2 cloves)

2 tbs. chopped fresh chives

1 teaspoon Dijon mustard

2 tbs. white wine vinegar

1/4 cup extra-virgin olive oil

salt and pepper

Directions:

1. Add everything to a large bowl.
2. Toss them well.
3. Serve.

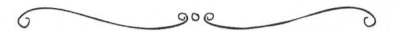

Cauliflower Sweet Potato Soup
Prep + Cook time: 15 minutes | Serves: 4

Nutritional Info (per serving)

Calories	Fat (g)	Protein (g)	Carbs (g)	Fiber (g)
230	6.3	6.8	26.3	0.3

Ingredients:

12 ounces cauliflower florets (frozen)

10 ounces sweet potato cubes (frozen)

1 red onion, chopped

1 fennel bulb, chopped

1 small fresh turmeric root, chopped (or 1 teaspoon ground)

1-inch fresh ginger, chopped

2 cloves garlic, chopped

sea salt and black pepper

4 cups of veggie broth or water

variety of chopped fresh herbs, for serving

Directions:

1. Add everything to the insert of an Instant Pot.
2. Fill the broth up to maximum limit of the pot.
3. Secure the lid and pressure cook the soup for 5 minutes.
4. Puree the cooked soup using a hand-heldblender.
5. Make sure to keep the soup chunky.
6. Garnish with chopped fresh herbs.
7. Serve warm.

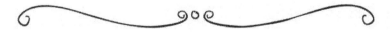

Artichoke Gazpacho

Prep + Cook time: 55 minutes | Serves: 6

Nutritional Info (per serving)

Calories	*Fat (g)*	*Protein (g)*	*Carbs (g)*	*Fiber (g)*
313	7.9	3.7	16.1	0.4

Ingredients:

30 whole artichoke hearts

3 ribs celery chopped

2 whole shallots chopped

4 cloves garlic chopped

3 tbs. olive oil divided

juice 1 lemon divided

1 bunch fresh thyme leaves only

sea salt and cracked black pepper

1/4 cup coconut cream unsweetened

4 cups vegetable broth

Directions:

1. Let your oven preheat at 375 degrees. Layer a baking sheet with aluminum foil.
2. Toss the artichoke hearts with garlic, shallots, and celery with salt, pepper, lemon juice, thyme and olive oil in a baking sheet.
3. Bake them for 55 minutes in the preheated oven.
4. Toss the veggies when baked halfway through.
5. Meanwhile, you can blend the coconut cream with broth in a blender.
6. Add the baked vegetables to the cream mixture.
7. Lightly puree this mixture then garnish with thyme, salt, and pepper.
8. Serve warm.

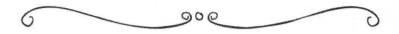

Fettuccine Noodles

Prep + Cook time: 15 minutes | Serves: 2

Nutritional Info (per serving)

Calories	Fat (g)	Protein (g)	Carbs (g)	Fiber (g)
241	0.4	2.7	17.1	0.2

Ingredients:

2 packs shirataki fettuccine noodles

3 tbs. olive oil, divided

Zest and juice of 1 lemon

3 garlic cloves, thinly sliced

1 bunch asparagus tips

1.5 cups asparagus stalks, thinly sliced

1 teaspoon of sea salt

1/4 teaspoon black pepper

Directions:

1. Prepare and cook the shirataki noodles for 2 minutes in boiling water.
2. Drain and keep them aside.
3. Preheat 2 tbsp oil in a suitable sauté pan.
4. Toss in garlic, asparagus, and lemon zest, stir cook for 5 minutes.
5. Now add noodles, salt, pepper, lemon juice, and remaining oil.
6. Stir cook for 4 minutes.
7. Garnish as desired.
8. Serve.

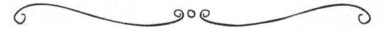

Sweet potato curry

Nutritional Info (per serving)

Calories	*Fat (g)*	*Protein (g)*	*Carbs (g)*	*Fiber (g)*
385	7.4	0.8	23.1	0.2

Ingredients:

1 tbsp coconut oil

1 onion, chopped

2 garlic cloves, grated

thumb-sized piece ginger, grated

3 tbsp Thai red curry paste

1 tbsp smooth almond butter

1 lb. sweet potato, peeled and cut into chunks

1 2/3 cup coconut milk

1 cup bag spinach

1 lime, juiced

cooked rice, to serve (optional)

Directions:

1. Add 1 tbsp coconut oil to a saucepan and heat it.
2. Stir in onion and sauté for 5 minutes.
3. Add garlic cloves, and ginger, stir cook for 2 minutes.
4. Now toss in curry paste, butter, and sweet potato.
5. Pour in water and coconut milk and let it cook on a simmer for 30 minutes.
6. Stir in lime juice, spinach, and more seasoning if needed.
7. Serve warm.

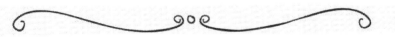

Arugula and Za'atar Pizza
Prep + Cook time: 25 minutes | Serves: 6

Nutritional Info (per serving)

Calories	Fat (g)	Protein (g)	Carbs (g)	Fiber (g)
250	0.7	4.6	18.1	0.2

Ingredients:

Dough:

½ cup of coconut milk

¼ cup coconut or avocado oil

1 cup arrowroot flour

¼ cup coconut flour

½ tsp sea salt

¼ tsp garlic powder

1 egg, whisked

Toppings:

Olive oil

1 tsp. za'atar

5-7 fresh basil leaves (optional)

A handful of arugula

3-4 oz. parmesan cheese, shredded

Juice from a ¼ lemon

Directions:

1. Let your oven preheat at 400 degrees F. Line a pizza pan with parchment paper.
2. Warm coconut milk with oil in a saucepan on medium heat.
3. Combine coconut flour, garlic powder, salt and arrowroot in a separate bowl.
4. Stir in the heated milk and mix well to form a smooth dough. Let it rest for 5 minutes.

5. Fold in whisk eggs and transfer the dough over a parchment paper.
6. Spread the dough with a spatula a thin as possible.
7. Bake this dough for 10 minutes then remove it from the oven.
8. Drizzle olive oil over the crust.
9. Spread a layer of za'atar, basil leaves, and parmesan cheese.
10. Bake again for 3 minutes.
11. Toss arugula with salt, pepper, lemon juice, and olive oil.
12. Spread the arugula over the pizza and bake again for 3 minutes.
13. Slice and serve.

Sprout Noodle Slaw
Prep + Cook time: 35 minutes | Serves: 1

Nutritional Info (per serving)

Calories	Fat (g)	Protein (g)	Carbs (g)	Fiber (g)
238	8	3.6	21.1	0.5

Ingredients:

4 ounces shirataki noodles

6 cups cabbage, shredded

½ pound (about 12) Brussels sprouts, shredded

4 carrots, peeled and chopped

1 bunch of green onions, chopped

Sesame dressing

3 tbs. white wine vinegar

3 tbs. toasted sesame oil

3 tbs. tamari

2 tbs. honey

½ cup almond butter

1 tbs. finely grated fresh ginger

2 garlic cloves, pressed

Garnish

A handful of cilantro, torn   1 lime, sliced into wedges

Optional, for spice lovers: sriracha or chili-garlic sauce

Directions:

1. Cook the noodles as per the instructions on the box.
2. Grate the vegetables either in a processor or using a knife.
3. Mix everything for the dressing a medium-sized bowl.
4. Stir in 1 tbs. water to the dressing. Adjust seasoning with salt.
5. Toss the noodles with grated vegetables and prepared dressing in a bowl.
6. Let It sit for 20 minutes in the refrigerator.
7. Garnish with lime wedges, cilantro, and sriracha.
8. Serve fresh.

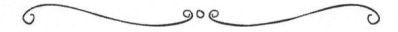

Thai Red Curry with Vegetables
Prep + Cook time: 25 minutes | Serves: 2

Nutritional Info (per serving)

Calories	*Fat (g)*	*Protein (g)*	*Carbs (g)*	*Fiber (g)*

Ingredients:

1 tbs. coconut oil or olive oil	2 tbs. Thai red curry paste
1 small white onion, chopped	1 can (14 ounces) coconut milk
Pinch of salt, more to taste	½ cup of water
1 tbs. ginger, grated	1 ½ cups packed thinly sliced kale
2 cloves garlic, pressed or minced	
1 zucchini, sliced	1 ½ teaspoon coconut sugar
4 carrots, peeled and sliced	1 tbs. tamari
	2 teaspoons fresh lime juice

Garnishes/sides: a handful of chopped fresh basil or cilantro

Directions:

1. Heat a greased skillet and sauté onion for 5 minutes.
2. Sprinkle salt over it then add garlic and ginger. Stir cook for 30 seconds.
3. Stir in carrots and zucchini. Sauté for 3 minutes then add curry paste.
4. Cook for 2 minutes then pour in water, coconut milk, sugar, and kale.
5. Let this mixture cook on a simmer for 10 minutes until veggies are soft.
6. Turn off the heat then adjust seasoning with salt, tamari, and lemon juice.
7. Serve warm.

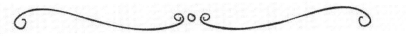

Kale and Coconut Rice

Prep + Cook time: 25 minutes | Serves: 3

Nutritional Info (per serving)

Calories	Fat (g)	Protein (g)	Carbs (g)	Fiber (g)
233	1.3	15	13.1	1.2

Ingredients:

2 tbs. coconut oil

2 pastured eggs, whisked

2 big cloves garlic, pressed or minced

¾ cup chopped green onions

1 cup chopped vegetables, like: Brussels sprouts or carrot

1 medium bunch kale, chopped

¼ teaspoon fine sea salt

¾ cup large, unsweetened coconut flakes

2 cups cooked and chilled cauliflower rice

2 teaspoons reduced-sodium tamari

2 teaspoons chili garlic sauce or sriracha

1 lime, halved

Handful fresh cilantro, for garnish

Directions:

1. Take a large skillet and heat a teaspoon of oil in it.
2. Add whisked eggs and stir cook for 2-3 minutes to make an egg scramble.
3. Transfer the scramble to a plate.
4. Heat more oil in the same pan and sauté green onion, garlic and other veggies in it.
5. Stir cook for 30 seconds then add kale and salt.

6. Cook more for 2 minutes then transfer this mixture to the eggs.
7. Heat about 2 teaspoons of oil in the same pan and stir cook coconut flakes for 30 secs.
8. Stir in rice and cook for another 3 minutes.
9. Transfer the rice to the scrambled eggs.
10. Stir in tamari, lime juice and garlic sauce.
11. Combine well the garnish with lime wedges, cilantro leaves.
12. Serve fresh.

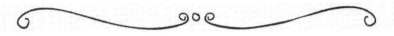

Farro Avocado Salad
Prep + Cook time: 55 minutes | Serves: 2

Nutritional Info (per serving)

Calories	*Fat (g)*	*Protein (g)*	*Carbs (g)*	*Fiber (g)*
279	6.8	4.1	22.9	1.2

Ingredients:

Roasted cauliflower

1 large head cauliflower (about 2 pounds), cut into bite-sized florets

¼ teaspoon black pepper

¼ teaspoon fine sea salt

2 tbs. extra-virgin olive oil
  For farro

1 cup uncooked farro, rinsed

2 cloves garlic, pressed or minced

2 teaspoons extra-virgin olive oil

¼ teaspoon fine sea salt

⅓ cup pitted Kalamata olives, rinsed, sliced

1 tbs. lemon juice (about ½ lemon), plus more for serving

Freshly ground black pepper, to taste

1 avocado, sliced into thin strips

4+ handfuls leafy greens

Directions:

1. Let your oven preheat at 425 degrees F.
2. Mix cauliflower with salt, pepper and olive oil.
3. Spread the florets in a baking sheet and roast them for 35 minutes.
4. Meanwhile, take a saucepan and cook the farro in 3 cups of water.
5. Let it cook on a simmer for 15 minutes then drain.
6. Mix it with salt, garlic and olive oil.
7. In a serving bowl, place cauliflower with olives, lemon juice, and cooked farro.
8. Garnish with avocado and greens.
9. Serve fresh.

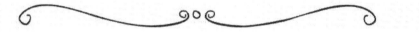

Cabbage Wraps with Crispy Tofu
Prep + Cook time: 45 minutes | Serves: 2

Nutritional Info (per serving)

Calories	*Fat (g)*	*Protein (g)*	*Carbs (g)*	*Fiber (g)*
215	1.7	7.3	16.3	0.5

Ingredients:

Crispy baked tofu

1 (15 ounces) block of organic extra-firm tofu

1 tbs. olive oil

1 tbs. reduced-sodium tamari or soy sauce

2 teaspoons arrowroot starch or cornstarch

Almond sauce

⅓ cup creamy almond butter

2 tbs. apple cider

2 tbs. tamari

2 tbs. honey

2 teaspoons toasted sesame oil

½ lime, juiced

2 garlic cloves, pressed or minced

Mango pico

2 ripe mangos, diced

½ bunch (about 4) green onions, chopped

⅓ cup packed fresh cilantro leaves, chopped

1 jalapeño, minced

½ lime, juiced

⅛ teaspoon salt

1 small head of green cabbage

2 tbs. large, unsweetened coconut flakes

Directions:

1. Let your oven preheat at 400 degrees F. Layer a baking sheet with wax paper.

2. Squeeze and drain the tofu then dice it down.
3. Prepare the sauce first by blending all of its ingredients in a blender.
4. Transfer the tofu cubes to a bowl, then toss in tamari and olive oil.
5. Drizzle 1 teaspoon arrowroot powder over them to coat well.
6. Transfer the tofu to a baking sheet. Bake them for 35 minutes.
7. Make sure to toss them when cooked half way through.
8. Combine everything for mango salsa in a bowl.
9. Spread the cabbage leaves on the serving plate.
10. Top them with baked tofu, almond sauce and coconut flakes.
11. Serve with mango salsa.
12. Serve.

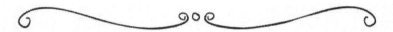

Salad and Sides Recipes

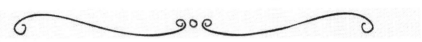

Caesar Salad

Prep + Cook time: 25 minutes | Serves: 4

Nutritional Info (per serving)

Calories	Fat (g)	Protein (g)	Carbs (g)	Fiber (g)
126	2.5	6.5	14.4	0.6

Ingredients:

1 large head romaine lettuce, chopped

2 small cloves of garlic, minced

5-6 tbsp extra virgin olive oil

2 tbsp lemon juice

2 tbsp nutritional yeast

1 tsp Dijon mustard

6 drops of liquid stevia

Heavy pinch of salt

Italian Crusted Tempeh

6 oz. tempeh, diced or sliced

2 tbsp olive oil

2 tsp nutritional yeast

1/4 tsp of truffle salt

1/4 tsp Italian seasoning

1/8 tsp black pepper

Directions:

1. Toss the tempeh with Italian seasoning, truffle salt, yeast, and black pepper to season well.
2. Now take a skillet and heat the olive oil in it.
3. Stir in the tempeh and sauté it for 3 minutes, until golden brown.
4. Meanwhile, mix rest of the ingredients in a large bowl.
5. Top the salad with the seared tempeh.
6. Serve fresh.

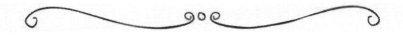

Lime Fruit Salad

Prep + Cook time: 15 minutes | Serves: 1

Nutritional Info (per serving)

Calories	*Fat (g)*	*Protein (g)*	*Carbs (g)*	*Fiber (g)*
255	1.5	4.7	16.4	1.3

Ingredients:

2/3 cup fresh orange juice

½ teaspoon orange zest

1/3 cup fresh lemon juice

½ teaspoon lemon zest

1 tbs. lime juice

Salad

½ teaspoon lime zest

¼ cup Swerve

1 teaspoon vanilla extract

1 teaspoon poppyseeds

1 can (15 ounces) mandarin oranges, thoroughly drained

2 cups fresh strawberries, hulled and sliced

3 kiwis, peeled, halved, and sliced

1 cup seedless grapes

1 cups blueberries

2 large mangoes, peeled and diced

1 cup blackberries

1 cup raspberries

Directions:

1. Combine all the zest and juices with sweetener in a saucepan and boil them.

2. Later let the mixture simmer for 5 minutes then toss in poppyseeds and vanilla extract. Allow this mixture to cool.
3. Prepare all the fruits and toss them gently together in a large salad bowl.
4. Pour in the prepared dressing and mix well.
5. Serve fresh.

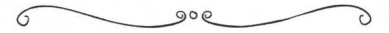

Kale Ginger Carrot Salad

Prep + Cook time: 15 minutes | Serves: 4

Nutritional Info (per serving)

Calories	*Fat (g)*	*Protein (g)*	*Carbs (g)*	*Fiber (g)*
106	3	6.2	23.4	1.6

Ingredients:

Salad:

3 cups kale leaves, finely chopped

2 cups finelychopped broccoli florets

2 cups finelychopped red cabbage

1 cup matchstick (shredded) carrots

1 cup roughlychopped fresh cilantro leaves

1/2 cup toasted slivered almonds

1/3 cup thinlysliced green onions

1 avocado, peeled pitted and diced

1 batch Carrot Ginger Dressing

Carrot- Dressing:

1 large carrot, peeled and roughly chopped

1/4 cup rice wine vinegar

2 tbs. avocado oil or olive oil

1 tbs. finelychopped fresh ginger

1 tbs. honey

1 tbs. white miso

1/2 teaspoon toasted sesame oil

Kosher salt and black pepper, to taste

Directions:

1. Add all the ingredients for dressing to the blender and pulse it until smooth.
2. Toss the remaining ingredients in a suitable salad bowl.
3. Pour in the prepared dressing.
4. Mix it all together gently using a spatula.
5. Serve fresh.

Avocado Tuna Salad
Prep + Cook time: 15 minutes | Serves: 4

Nutritional Info (per serving)

Calories	Fat (g)	Protein (g)	Carbs (g)	Fiber (g)
176	8.5	3.5	6.4	2.6

Ingredients

15 oz tuna in oil, drained and flaked

1 English cucumber sliced

3 medium avocados peeled, pitted and sliced

1 small red onion thinly sliced

1/4 cup cilantro

2 Tbsp lemon juice freshly squeezed

2 Tbsp extra virgin olive oil

1 tsp sea salt or to taste

1/8 tsp black pepper

Directions:

1. Toss cucumber, onion, tuna, avocado and cilantro in a bowl.
2. Stir in lemon juice, salt, pepper, and olive oil.
3. Mix well gently with a spatula.
4. Serve fresh.

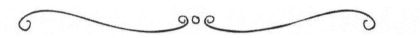

Chicken, Avocado Salad

Prep + Cook time: 25 minutes | Serves: 2

Nutritional Info (per serving)

Calories	*Fat (g)*	*Protein (g)*	*Carbs (g)*	*Fiber (g)*
134	8.5	13.5	3.4	2.1

Ingredients:

1 pound boneless skinless chicken tenders

1/4 cup extra virgin olive oil

4 cloves garlic, minced or grated

1/4 cup fresh parsley, chopped

1/4 cup fresh basil, chopped

1/2 teaspoon smoked paprika

1/2 teaspoon onion powder

1/4 teaspoon cayenne

1/2 teaspoon kosher salt and pepper

2 heads romaine lettuce, chopped

1 cup fresh strawberries, halved

2 watermelon radishes, thinly sliced

2 Persian cucumbers, sliced

4 ounces herbed goat cheese, crumbled

1 avocado, sliced

1/2 cup roasted almonds, chopped

Directions:

1. Season the chicken with garlic, olive oil, parsley, onion powder, salt, pepper, cayenne, paprika and basil in a bowl.
2. Cover the seasoned chicken and let it marinate overnight or atleast 1 hour.
3. Lit up the grill and preheat it on medium heat.
4. Grease its grilling grates and grill the chicken for 5 minutes per side.
5. Place the grilled chicken on the cutting board and slice it into pieces.
6. Toss the remaining ingredients in a suitable salad bowl.
7. Mix well then top the salad with chicken slices.
8. Serve fresh.

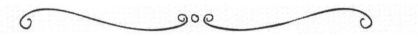

Grilled Romaine Chicken Salad
Prep + Cook time: 25 minutes | Serves: 4

Nutritional Info (per serving)

Calories	Fat (g)	Protein (g)	Carbs (g)	Fiber (g)
151	4	17.5	13	1.3

Ingredients

Dressing:

½ lime, juice   4 teaspoons olive oil

1/2 cup jarred mild salsa

For Chicken

4 boneless, chicken thighs   1/4 teaspoon dried oregano

3/4 teaspoon kosher salt   1/4 teaspoon cumin

For Grilled Salad

2 romaine hearts   2 tbs. diced red onion

olive oil spray   pinch of kosher salt

4 oz. avocado (1 small has) sliced

Directions:

1. Season the chicken with salt, cumin and oregano in a bowl.
2. Cover the seasoned chicken and marinate it for 1 hour.
3. Lit up the grill and preheat it on medium heat.
4. Grease its grilling grates and grill the chicken for 5 minutes per side.
5. Place the grilled chicken on the cutting board and slice it into pieces.
6. Grill the romaine hearts and onion in the grill for 2-3 minutes.
7. Toss the remaining ingredients in a suitable salad bowl.
8. Add the grilled chicken, romaine hearts, and onion to the bowl.
9. Serve fresh.

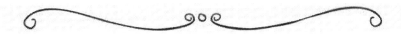

Avocado Spinach Salad with Chicken
Prep + Cook time: 45 minutes | Serves: 2

Nutritional Info (per serving)

Calories	*Fat (g)*	*Protein (g)*	*Carbs (g)*	*Fiber (g)*
133	7.3	11	8.4	1.4

Ingredients:

1/4 cup extra virgin olive oil

1 tbs. golden balsamic vinegar

1 teaspoon swerve

1 tbs. roughly chopped fresh tarragon

1/4 teaspoon kosher salt

1/4 teaspoon freshly ground black pepper

2 boneless skinless chicken breasts

6 cups loosely packed fresh spinach

6-8 large strawberries hulled and quartered

1 avocado peeled, seeded and diced

3-4 thinly sliced rings of red onion

2 tbs. sliced almonds

Directions:

1. Combine olive oil with sweetener, tarragon, vinegar, salt and pepper in a bowl.
2. Season the chicken with half of the dressing and cover it to marinate for 30 mins.
3. Grease a grill pan and sear the chicken for 3 minutes per side.

4. Cook the chicken on low heat for 25 minutes while flipping after every 5 minutes.
5. Toss the remaining ingredients in a suitable salad bowl.
6. Slice the cooked chicken and toss it into the salad.
7. Add avocado sliced and almond to the salad.
8. Serve fresh.

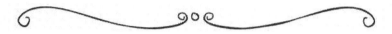

Broccoli Spinach Salad
Prep + Cook time: 15 minutes | Serves: 4

Nutritional Info (per serving)

Calories	Fat (g)	Protein (g)	Carbs (g)	Fiber (g)
216	5.5	6	13.1	1.2

Ingredients:

4 oz. fresh baby spinach

1/2 cup chopped broccoli

1/2 a ripe avocado

1/4 cup blueberries

1/4 cup crumbled feta cheese

2-4 TBSP dried cranberries

2-4 TBSP roasted sunflower seeds

black pepper to taste (optional)

POPPY SEED RANCH DRESSING:

1/2 cup of greek yogurt

1/4 cup almond milk

1/4 cup lectin free mayonnaise

1 clove ground

1/2 tsp lemon juice

1 tsp poppy seeds

1/2 tsp dried parsley

1/2 tsp dill, dried

1/4 tsp onion powder ground

1/4 tsp paprika

1/8-1/4 tsp garlic powder to taste

1/8 tsp sea salt

1/8 tsp black pepper

Directions:

1. Whisk all the ingredients for dressing in a salad bowl.
2. Toss in the remaining ingredients.
3. Serve fresh.

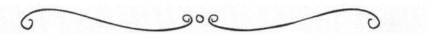

Sweet Potato Quinoa Salad
Prep + Cook time: 25 minutes | Serves: 4

Nutritional Info (per serving)

Calories	Fat (g)	Protein (g)	Carbs (g)	Fiber (g)
144	3.1	8.2	27.1	1.4

Ingredients:

2 medium sweet potatoes, peeled and chopped

1 and 1/2 tbs. olive oil

Sea salt and black pepper, to taste

1 cup quinoa uncooked

2 cups of water

4-5 ounces fresh spinach, chopped

1 large avocado, chopped

1/3 cup dried cranberries

Lemon Vinaigrette

4 tbs. red wine vinegar

1 and 1/2 tbs. Dijon mustard

1/2 teaspoon dried oregano

1 teaspoon dried basil

1 clove garlic, minced

1/2 cup olive oil

3 tbs. juice

Directions:

1. Let your oven preheat at 425 degrees F. Toss the potatoes with salt, pepper and olive oil in a baking sheet.
2. Roast the potatoes for 15 minutes then toss them well.
3. Return the potatoes to the oven and bake again for 20 minutes.
4. Meanwhile, cook the quinoa in the water in a covered pan until al dente.
5. Fluff the cooked quinoa and transfer it to the salad bowl.
6. Turn off the heat and let rest covered for 5 minutes.
7. Remove the lid after 5 minutes then fluff the quinoa with a fork.
8. Toss the cooked quinoa and sweet potato in a large bowl.
9. Stir in all the remaining ingredients and mix them well.
10. Enjoy.

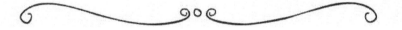

Pistachio Greens salad
Prep + Cook time: 15 minutes | Serves: 6

Nutritional Info (per serving)

Calories	*Fat (g)*	*Protein (g)*	*Carbs (g)*	*Fiber (g)*
154	4.2	16	21.4	1.3

Ingredients

4-6 cups greens, chopped

1 green apple, chopped

1 cup chopped cucumber

1 cup shelled edamame

1/2 cup green onion, thinly sliced

1 avocado, chopped

1 cup broccoli, cut in florets

1 cup green grapes, cut in half

1/2 cup pistachios, roughly chopped

Herb Dressing:

1/3 cup olive oil

Juice of 1 lemon

1/2 teaspoon dijon mustard

1/2 teaspoon erythritol syrup

2 tbs. chopped fresh herbs, your favorite kind

1 small clove garlic, minced

1/4 teaspoon salt

1/8 teaspoon black pepper

Directions:

1. Combine all the ingredients for dressing in a salad bowl.
2. Toss in all the remaining ingredients to the bowl.
3. Mix gently and enjoy.

Chicken Salad with Honey

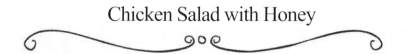

Vinaigrette

Prep + Cook time: 15 minutes | Serves: 4

Nutritional Info (per serving)

Calories	Fat (g)	Protein (g)	Carbs (g)	Fiber (g)
152	4.1	14.5	7.1	0.7

Ingredients:

5 cups romaine lettuce, chopped

1 cup arugula

1 boneless chicken breast, cooked and chopped

5 slices of bacon, cooked and chopped

2 hard-boiled pastured eggs, peeled and sliced

2 apples, sliced

1 avocado, sliced

½ cup walnuts, chopped

Honey Apple Cider Dressing:

¾ cup olive oil

¾ cup apple cider vinegar

2 tbs. water

¼ cup honey

1 teaspoon salt

¼ teaspoon pepper

Directions:

1. Mix all the ingredients for dressing in a salad bowl.
2. Toss in the remaining ingredients and mix gently.
3. Enjoy.

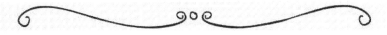

Chopped Thai Salad

Prep + Cook time: 25 minutes | Serves: 4

Nutritional Info (per serving)

Calories	*Fat (g)*	*Protein (g)*	*Carbs (g)*	*Fiber (g)*
137	2.5	0.6	14.8	3.2

Ingredients:

3 cups finely shredded cabbage

1/2 cup cucumbers, chopped

For the dressing:

1/3 cup almond butter

1 tbs. soy sauce

1 tbs. honey

1 tbs. lime juice

1 cup shelled edamame

1/2 cup carrots, shredded or julienned

2 tbs. chopped cilantro

2 teaspoons sesame oil

1 teaspoon chili garlic sauce

3 tbs. warm water

Directions:

1. Mix all the ingredients for dressing in a salad bowl.
2. Toss in the remaining ingredients and mix gently.
3. Enjoy.

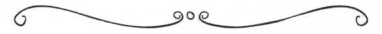

Avocado Spiralized Cucumber Salad

Prep + Cook time: 15 minutes | Serves: 4

Nutritional Info (per serving)

Calories	Fat (g)	Protein (g)	Carbs (g)	Fiber (g)
141	0.3	0.6	13.2	0.6

Ingredients:

2 cucumber peeled and spiralized

6.5oz wild caught crab meat (fresh or canned), drained

2 tbsp chopped cilantro

¼ teaspoon black pepper

1/2 tsp minced garlic

2 tsp sesame oil (divided)

2 tsp rice vinegar

splash of lime

1 whole avocado (sliced or chopped)

1 large plum

sesame seeds (optional)

sea salt / black pepper to taste

Directions:

1. Mix all the ingredients for dressing in a salad bowl.
2. Toss in the remaining ingredients and mix gently.
3. Enjoy.

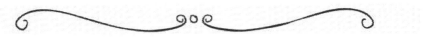

Zucchini Mexican Salad
Prep + Cook time: 25 minutes | Serves: 4

Nutritional Info (per serving)

Calories	Fat (g)	Protein (g)	Carbs (g)	Fiber (g)
149	0.4	0.5	11.5	0.9

Ingredients

3 zucchini ends cut off and halved

1 carrot, cut in chunks

2 tbs. olive oil

1 small jalapeno pepper, deseeded, charred and peeled.

1/4 cup minced fresh cilantro

Dressing

1/4 cup lime juice

1 tbs. Dijon mustard

1 tbs. agave syrup

2 tbs. minced fresh cilantro

1/4 cup olive oil

Salt and pepper to taste

Directions:

1. Mix all the ingredients for dressing in a salad bowl.
2. Lit up the grill and preheat it on medium heat.
3. Charr and grill all the vegetables for 4 minutes per sides.
4. Make sure to brush the veggies with olive oil while grilling
5. Transfer them to the salad bowl and mix gently.
6. Enjoy.

Crunchy Avocado Salads

Prep + Cook time: 15 minutes | Serves: 2

Nutritional Info (per serving)

Calories	Fat (g)	Protein (g)	Carbs (g)	Fiber (g)
175	1.6	3.8	13.4	1.3

Ingredients:

2 cups fresh arugula

1/2 avocado pitted and sliced

3 slices fresh mozzarella cheese

fresh basil leaves

1 tbs. extra-virgin olive oil

1 1/2 teaspoons balsamic vinegar

1 dollop of honey

kosher salt and freshly ground black pepper

Directions:

1. Mix all the ingredients for dressing in a salad bowl.
2. Toss in the remaining ingredients and mix gently.
3. Enjoy.

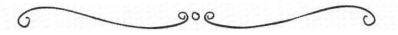

Tahini Kale Salad

Prep + Cook time: 15 minutes | Serves: 4

Nutritional Info (per serving)

Calories	Fat (g)	Protein (g)	Carbs (g)	Fiber (g)
128	3.3	13.8	23.4	1.4

Ingredients:

Dressing:

2 limes juiced

zest of 1 lime

2 tbs. fishsauce

2 tbs. ponzu sauce

2-3 tbs. sweet Thai chili sauce

1-2 cloves garlic minced or grated

1 tbs. fresh ginger grated

2-3 tbs. tahini

SALAD:

4 cups baby kale or other dark leafy green

1-ounce bag frozen shelled edamame defrosted and cooked

4 carrots shredded

1 cup fresh mango, chopped

2 lemongrass stalks, chopped

4 green onions chopped

3/4 cups of fresh basil and cilantro

4 hard-boiledpastured eggs diced

1/4 cup black and/or white sesame seeds toasted

Directions:

1. Mix all the ingredients for dressing in a salad bowl.
2. Toss in the remaining ingredients and mix gently.
3. Enjoy.

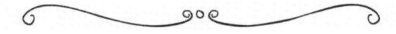

Roasted Asparagus Salad
Prep + Cook time: 35 minutes | Serves: 4

Nutritional Info (per serving)

Calories	*Fat (g)*	*Protein (g)*	*Carbs (g)*	*Fiber (g)*
109	0.3	4.7	9	1.4

Ingredients

1 whole bunch of fresh asparagus, trimmed and cut into chunks

2-3 tbs. avocado oil

1 pinch garlic powder, or to taste

4 cups lettuce leaves, cut into bite-size pieces

1 cup olives, halved

Directions:

1. Toss asparagus with avocado oil and garlic powder in a baking sheet.
2. Bake the asparagus for 20 minutes in the preheated oven at 400 degrees F.
3. Mix the asparagus with remaining ingredients in a salad bowl.
4. Serve.

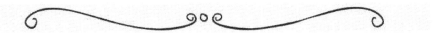

Strawberry Spinach Salad

Prep + Cook time: 15 minutes | Serves: 4

Nutritional Info (per serving)

Calories	*Fat (g)*	*Protein (g)*	*Carbs (g)*	*Fiber (g)*
171	8	5.5	14	1.2

Ingredients:

2 tbs. sesame seeds

1 tbs. poppy seeds

1/2 cup Swerve

1/2 cup olive oil

1/4 cup distilled white vinegar

1/4 teaspoon paprika

1/4 teaspoon Worcestershire sauce

1 tbs. minced onion

10 ounces fresh spinach, rinsed, dried and torn

1-quart strawberries, cleaned, hulled and sliced

1/4 cup almonds, blanched and slivered

Directions:

1. Mix all the ingredients for dressing in a salad bowl.
2. Toss in the remaining ingredients and mix gently.
3. Enjoy.

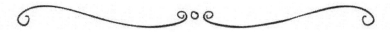

Asparagus, Orange and Endive Salad
Prep + Cook time: 15 minutes | Serves: 4

Nutritional Info (per serving)

Calories	Fat (g)	Protein (g)	Carbs (g)	Fiber (g)
132	8.3	3.1	12.2	3.3

Ingredients:

2 1/2 cups asparagus, diagonally sliced

2 cups rinsed, dried and torn endive leaves

2 large oranges, sliced into rounds

1 red onion, thinly sliced

1/3 cup raspberry vinegar

2 tbs. canola oil

1 tbs. orange juice

1 tbs. swerve

salt and pepper to taste

Directions:

1. Add sliced asparagus to boiling water for 1 minute then immediately drain it.
2. Rinse under cold water and keep it aside.
3. Toss the blanched asparagus with onion, endive, oranges, and endive.
4. Stir in the remaining ingredients then mix well gently.
5. Serve fresh.

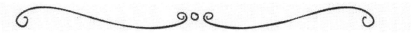

Chicken Salad with Spicy Dressing
Prep + Cook time: 15 minutes | Serves: 4

Nutritional Info (per serving)

Calories	Fat (g)	Protein (g)	Carbs (g)	Fiber (g)
143	7.6	16.1	4.3	0.8

Ingredients:

1/2 cup almond butter, melted

1 tbs. sambal oelek

1 tbs. soy sauce, low sodium

1 teaspoon toasted sesame oil

4 tbs. water, or more as needed

1 cucumber, peeled and sliced into thin strips

1 cooked chicken breast, shredded into thin strands

Directions:

1. Mix all the ingredients for dressing in a salad bowl.
2. Toss in the remaining ingredients and mix gently.

3. Enjoy.

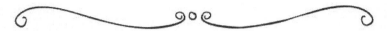

Cranberry Spinach Salad
Prep + Cook time: 15 minutes | Serves: 4

Nutritional Info (per serving)

Calories	*Fat (g)*	*Protein (g)*	*Carbs (g)*	*Fiber (g)*
161	3.6	3.7	22.3	1.3

Ingredients:

1 tbs almond butter, melted

3/4 cup almonds, blanched

1 pound spinach, rinsed and torn into pieces

1 cup dried cranberries

2 tbs toasted sesame seeds

1 tbs poppy seeds

1/2 cup Swerve

2 tbs minced onion

1/4 teaspoon paprika

1/4 cup white wine vinegar

1/4 cup cider vinegar

1/2 cup vegetable oil

Directions:

1. Mix all the ingredients for dressing in a salad bowl.
2. Toss in the remaining ingredients and mix gently.
3. Enjoy.

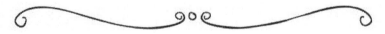

Mediterranean Greek Salad
Prep + Cook time: 15 minutes | Serves: 2

Nutritional Info (per serving)

Calories	Fat (g)	Protein (g)	Carbs (g)	Fiber (g)
113	4.4	0.9	0.4	1.4

Ingredients:

3 cucumbers, seeded and sliced

1 1/2 cups parmesan cheese

1 cup black olives, pitted and sliced

1/2 red onion, sliced

Salt and pepper, to taste

2 teaspoon lemon juice

Directions:

1. Mix all the ingredients for dressing in a salad bowl.
2. Toss in the remaining ingredients and mix gently.
3. Enjoy.

Broccoli Salad

Prep + Cook time: 15 minutes | Serves: 4

Nutritional Info (per serving)

Calories	Fat (g)	Protein (g)	Carbs (g)	Fiber (g)
118	1.7	13.5	8.6	1

Ingredients:

10 slices bacon

1 head fresh broccoli, cut into pieces

1/4 cup red onion, chopped

1/2 cup raisins

3 tbs white wine vinegar

2 tbs. swerve

1 cup sunflower seeds

1 cup lectin free mayonnaise

Directions:

1. Sauté bacon in a deep skillet for 5 minutes until crispy.
2. Drain the bacon and crumble it. keep it aside.
3. Mix all the ingredients for dressing in a salad bowl.
4. Toss in the remaining ingredients and mix gently.
5. Enjoy.

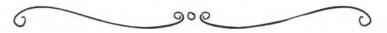

Cucumber Onion Salad

Prep + Cook time: 15 minutes | Serves: 2

Nutritional Info (per serving)

Calories	*Fat (g)*	*Protein (g)*	*Carbs (g)*	*Fiber (g)*
118	0.7	2.6	10.4	4.3

Ingredients:

4 cucumbers, thinly sliced

1 small white onion, thinly sliced

1 cup white vinegar

1/2 cup water

3/4 cup Swerve

1 tbs dried dill, or to taste

Directions:

1. Mix all the ingredients for dressing in a salad bowl.
2. Toss in the remaining ingredients and mix gently.
3. Enjoy.

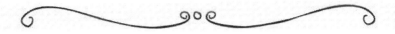

Thai Cucumber Salad

Prep + Cook time: 15 minutes | Serves: 4

Nutritional Info (per serving)

Calories	Fat (g)	Protein (g)	Carbs (g)	Fiber (g)
109	0.4	6.1	17.2	0.6

Ingredients:

3 large English cucumbers, peeled and cut into slices

1 tbs. salt

1/2 cup Swerve

1/2 cup rice wine vinegar

2 jalapeno peppers, seeded and chopped

1/4 cup chopped cilantro

Directions:

1. Place the cucumber in a suitablecolander and sprinkle salt over it.
2. Leave the cucumber for 30 minutes then drain it.
3. Mix all the ingredients for dressing in a salad bowl.
4. Toss in the remaining ingredients and mix gently.
5. Enjoy.

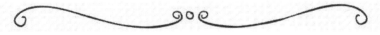

Amish Slaw

Prep + Cook time: 15 minutes | Serves: 2

Nutritional Info (per serving)

Calories	Fat (g)	Protein (g)	Carbs (g)	Fiber (g)
176	8.5	3.5	6.4	2.6

Ingredients:

1 medium head cabbage, cored and shredded

1 medium onion, finely chopped

1 cup Swerve

1 cup vinegar

1 teaspoon salt

1 teaspoon celery seed

1 teaspoon prepared mustard

3/4 cup vegetable oil

Directions:

1. Cook onion, cabbage, and sweetener in a saucepan, to a boil.
2. Add the remaining ingredients and cook for 3 minutes.
3. Allow it to cool then refrigerate for 1 hour.
4. Mix well and serve.

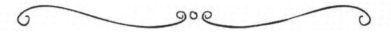

Sunday Fruit Salad

Prep + Cook time: 15 minutes | Serves: 4

Nutritional Info (per serving)

Calories	*Fat (g)*	*Protein (g)*	*Carbs (g)*	*Fiber (g)*
203	5	2.4	12	0.8

Ingredients

1 (20 ounces) can pineapple chunks

1 cup pineapple juice

2 apples, peeled and cored

1 (21 ounces) can peach pie filling

2 bananas, peeled and diced   1-pint strawberries

3 kiwis

Directions:

1. Soak apples in pineapple juice in a bowl for 10 minutes.
2. Toss peach pie filling with pineapple in a salad bowl,
3. Remove the soaked apples from the juice and add to the salad bowl.
4. Now add a banana to the same pineapple juice. Let it rest for 10 minutes.
5. Transfer the banana to the salad and add the remaining ingredients.
6. Mix well gently and serve.

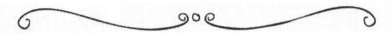

Green Salad with Cranberry Vinaigrette
Prep + Cook time: 5 minutes | Serves: 4

Nutritional Info (per serving)

Calories	*Fat (g)*	*Protein (g)*	*Carbs (g)*	*Fiber (g)*
132	1.6	3.7	10.4	0.2

Ingredients:

1 cup sliced almonds

3 tbs. red wine vinegar

1/3 cup olive oil

1/4 cup fresh cranberries

1 tbs. Dijon mustard

1/2 teaspoon minced garlic

1/2 teaspoon salt

1/2 teaspoon ground black pepper

2 tbs. water

1/2 red onion, thinly sliced

1 pound mixed salad greens

Directions:

1. Let your oven preheat at 375 degrees F.
2. Spread almonds in a baking sheet and roast them for 5 minutes in the oven.
3. Toss the almonds with green, and onion in a salad bowl.
4. Blend the remaining ingredients then pour it into the salad bowl.
5. Toss them well together.
6. Serve fresh.

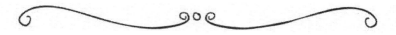

Spinach Cranberry Salad
Prep + Cook time: 5 minutes | Serves: 2

Nutritional Info (per serving)

Calories	*Fat (g)*	*Protein (g)*	*Carbs (g)*	*Fiber (g)*
104	3.6	1.4	9.6	1.3

Ingredients:

8 cups baby spinach leaves

1/2 medium red onion, sliced and rings separated

1 (11 ounces) can mandarin oranges, drained

1 1/2 cups sweetened dried cranberries

1 cup honey-roasted sliced almonds

1 cup balsamic vinaigrette salad dressing

Directions:

1. Mix all the ingredients for dressing in a salad bowl.
2. Toss in the remaining ingredients and mix gently.
3. Enjoy.

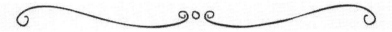

Cucumber Sunomono
Prep + Cook time: 5 minutes | Serves: 1

Nutritional Info (per serving)

Calories	*Fat (g)*	*Protein (g)*	*Carbs (g)*	*Fiber (g)*
76	0	0.5	1.3	1

Ingredients:

2 large cucumbers, peeled and seeds removed, sliced

1/3 cup rice vinegar

4 teaspoons swerve

1 teaspoon salt

1 1/2 teaspoons fresh ginger root, minced

Directions:

1. Mix all the ingredients for dressing in a salad bowl.
2. Toss in the remaining ingredients and mix gently.
3. Enjoy.

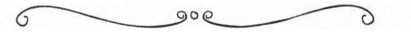

Dips and Sauces Recipes

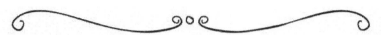

Hungarian Barbecue Sauce

Prep + Cook time: 35 minutes | Serves: 12

Nutritional Info (per serving)

Calories	Fat (g)	Protein (g)	Carbs (g)	Fiber (g)
23	0.5	1	4.3	0

Ingredients:

1/2 medium red onion, finely chopped

3 garlic cloves, smashed and finely chopped

3 anchovies' fillets, briefly rinsed

2 teaspoons avocado oil

1/4 teaspoon allspice

1/4 teaspoon turmeric powder

1/2 teaspoon mustard powder

1 teaspoon Hungarian paprika

1/2 teaspoon smoked Hungarian paprika

1/2 teaspoon cayenne pepper

1/2 teaspoon Tabasco

1 teaspoon apple cider vinegar

1/2 teaspoon monk fruit sweetener

1/4 teaspoon fresh ground pepper

Water

Directions:

1. Sauté onion, anchovies, and garlic with cooking oil in a pan until soft.
2. Stir in cider, sweetener, and spices, let it cook on low simmer for 20 mins.

3. Once cooked, transfer the sautéed mixture to the blender.
4. Puree this mixture, return the sauce to the pan.
5. Reheat the sauce to a boil then allow it to cool.
6. Serve or preserve in a clean jar.

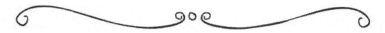

Sweet Potato Marinara
Prep + Cook time: 15 minutes | Serves: 12

Nutritional Info (per serving)

Calories	*Fat (g)*	*Protein (g)*	*Carbs (g)*	*Fiber (g)*
46	0.7	0.3	21.1	0.4

Ingredients:

1 cup dry red wine

1 15-ounce can sweet potato purée

3/4 cup coconut cream

1/4 cup fresh basil leaves, chopped

1/4 cup fresh parsley leaves, chopped

1/4 cup gratedparmesan cheese

Directions:

1. Warm up the sweet potato in a saucepan on medium heat.
2. Stir in parsley, and basil then let it cook for 2 mins.
3. Add cream and wine to the thick mixture.
4. After boiling the sauce, cook it for 8 minutes on a simmer.
5. Stir in parmesan and mix it well.

6. Serve.

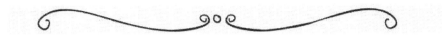

Carrot Based Marinara
Prep + Cook time: 45 minutes | Serves: 12

Nutritional Info (per serving)

Calories	*Fat (g)*	*Protein (g)*	*Carbs (g)*	*Fiber (g)*
12	0.4	0.1	1.2	0.2

Ingredients:

1 tbs. coconut oil

2 yellow onions, chopped

4 garlic cloves, minced

1-pound carrots, chopped

1 medium beet, chopped

1 cup of water

1 teaspoon of sea salt

2 tbs. fresh lemon juice

Directions:

1. Warm up the coconut oil in a stock pot on medium heat.
2. Add onions, sauté for 10 minutes.
3. Toss in garlic and stir cook for 1 minute.
4. Add water, carrots, and beet. Then cook it on a simmer for 40 minutes.
5. Once done, puree this mixture in a blender along with lemon juice and salt.
6. Add basil and oregano to the sauce.
7. Mix well and serve.

Coconut Pesto Sauce
Prep + Cook time: 15 minutes | Serves: 12

Nutritional Info (per serving)

Calories	Fat (g)	Protein (g)	Carbs (g)	Fiber (g)
19	1.1	0.9	2.1	0.3

Ingredients:

3 tbs. of almond butter

1/2 cup of full-fat coconut milk

1 cup of jarred or homemade pesto

4 ounces of grated parmesan

Sea salt, to taste

Cracked black pepper, to taste

Directions:

1. Warm up the coconut milk in a stock pot along with butter.
2. Stir in pesto, salt, black pepper, cheese, and red pepper.
3. Let it cookon a simmer, on low heat for 3 minutes.
4. Mix well and allow it to cool.
5. Serve.

Tabasco BBQ Sauce
Prep + Cook time: 25 minutes | Serves: 12

Nutritional Info (per serving)

Calories	Fat (g)	Protein (g)	Carbs (g)	Fiber (g)
13	1.3	0.5	1.8	0.1

Ingredients:

1 tbs. extra-virgin olive oil

2 cloves garlic finely minced

2 tbs. red onion finely minced

1 cup tomato sauce

1/4 cup apple cider vinegar

1 tbs. chipotle tabasco

1 tbs. lemon juice

1 tbs. raw local honey

1/2 tbs. ground mustard

1 teaspoon pure liquid smoke

1/2 teaspoon salt

1/2 teaspoon pepper

Directions:

1. Add olive oil to a stockpot and sauté garlic and onion in the pot until soft.
2. Toss in rest of the ingredients and let it simmer for 15 minutes on low heat after covering the lid.
3. Mix well and allow it cool.
4. Serve and preserve for later use.

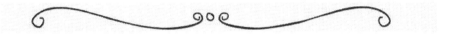

Buffalo Dip

Prep + Cook time: 55 minutes | Serves: 12

Nutritional Info (per serving)

Calories	Fat (g)	Protein (g)	Carbs (g)	Fiber (g)
17	1.3	0.2	6.8	0.1

Ingredients:

1 1/4 lbs. chicken tenders, boneless

1 tbs. olive oil

1/2 medium onion chopped

2 cloves garlic minced

1 tbs.avocado oil

2/3 cup paleo mayo

2/3 cup coconut cream

1 tbs. brown mustard

1 teaspoon garlic powder

1 teaspoon onion powder

1 teaspoon dried dill

1/2 teaspoon smoked paprika

1/3 cup hot sauce

1 1/2 tbs. fresh lemon juice

Directions:

1. Let your oven preheat at 400 degrees F and layer a baking sheet with a foil.
2. Place the chicken in the sheet and drizzle olive oil, pepper, and salt over it.
3. Bake it for 20 minutes in the preheated oven.
4. Lower down the oven temperature to 350 degrees F.
5. Add cooking oil to a skillet and sauté onion in it until soft.
6. Toss in garlic and cook for 30 seconds then remove it from the heat.
7. Whisk coconut cream, garlic powder, dill, onion powder, mayo, hot sauce, paprika, and lemon juice until creamy and smooth.
8. Shred the cooked chicken and toss it into the creamy mixture.
9. Fold in onion and garlic mixture.
10. Transfer this dip to a casserole dish and place in the oven for 25 minutes.
11. Serve fresh.

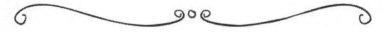

BBQ Ranch Dip
Prep + Cook time: 5 minutes | Serves: 12

Nutritional Info (per serving)

Calories	Fat (g)	Protein (g)	Carbs (g)	Fiber (g)
22	1.5	0.6	6.3	0.7

Ingredients:

1 medjool date pitted and softened

1 tbs. water

1/4 cup tomato sauce

3 tbs apple cider vinegar

1 teaspoon spicy brown mustard

1/2 cup homemade mayo, lectin free

1 teaspoon garlic powder

1 1/2 teaspoon onion powder

1 teaspoon smoked paprika

2 teaspoon dried chives

Salt and black pepper to taste

Dash cayenne pepper for spice optional

Directions:

1. Toss everything into the blender.
2. Pulse them well until smooth.
3. Serve fresh.

Chicken Spinach Dip
Prep + Cook time: 45 minutes | Serves: 8

Nutritional Info (per serving)

Calories	Fat (g)	Protein (g)	Carbs (g)	Fiber (g)
27	1.8	12.6	1.4	0.6

Ingredients:

1 lb. Chicken breasts or tenderloins

1 tbs olive or avocado oil

Salt and pepper to season chicken

1 tbs. coconut oil

1 medium onion chopped

3-4 cloves garlic finely chopped

Sea salt

10 oz. fresh baby spinach chopped

14 oz can artichoke hearts, drained and chopped

2/3 cup coconut cream

½ tbs lectin free mayo

1 tbs lemon juice

3 tbs nutritional yeast

1/2 teaspoon sea salt

Black pepper to taste

Directions:

1. Let your oven preheat at 400 degrees F.
2. Layer a baking sheet with wax paper and place the chicken in it.
3. Drizzle oil, pepper, and salt over it then bake for 25 minutes.
4. Add the coconut oil to a saucepan and sauté onion until soft.
5. Stir in garlic and cook for 1 minute.
6. Toss in spinach and artichoke cook until it is wilted. Turn off the heat.
7. Whisk lemon juice, yeast, salt, pepper, mayo, and cream in a bowl until smooth.
8. Shred the cooked chicken and transfer it to the creamy mixture.
9. Fold in spinach mixture then pour the dip into a casserole dish.
10. Bake it for 15 minutes then allow it to cool.
11. Serve fresh.

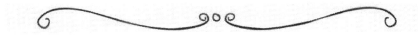

Cherry BBQ Sauce

Prep + Cook time: 5 minutes | Serves: 12

Nutritional Info (per serving)

Calories	Fat (g)	Protein (g)	Carbs (g)	Fiber (g)
13	0.2	0.3	1.3	0.5

Ingredients:

6 oz. organic tomato sauce

3/4 cup tart cherry juice

1 tbs blackstrap molasses

2 tbs apple cider vinegar

1 and 1/2 teaspoon liquid smoke

1/2 teaspoon onion powder

1/2 teaspoon smoked paprika

1/8-1/4 teaspoon chipotle pepper

dash sea salt

Directions:

1. Toss everything into the blender.
2. Pulse them well until smooth.
3. Serve fresh.

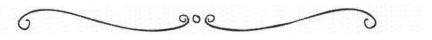

Chipotle Ketchup

Prep + Cook time: 5 minutes | Serves: 12

Nutritional Info (per serving)

Calories	Fat (g)	Protein (g)	Carbs (g)	Fiber (g)

| 16 | 0.4 | 2.1 | 14.1 | 0.3 |

Ingredients:

6 oz. organic tomato sauce

2 tbs. pure erythritol syrup

2 tbs. apple cider vinegar

1 teaspoon smoked paprika

1/2 teaspoon salt

1/4 teaspoon chipotle Chile

2 tbs. water

1/2 teaspoon onion powder

Directions:

1. Toss everything into the blender.
2. Pulse them well until smooth.
3. Serve fresh.

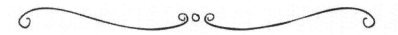

Chili Garlic Paste

Prep + Cook time: 35 minutes | Serves: 8

Nutritional Info (per serving)

Calories	*Fat (g)*	*Protein (g)*	*Carbs (g)*	*Fiber (g)*
10	0	0	3.3	0.1

Ingredients:

1 lb. red Fresno peppers, peeled and deseeded	2 teaspoon apple cider vinegar
4-6 tbs. of water	1 teaspoon erythritol
3 large garlic cloves, smashed	1/4 teaspoon salt
	1/8 teaspoon onion powder

Directions:

1. Let your oven preheat at 500 degrees F.
2. Deseed the sliced chilis then place them in a baking sheet.
3. Roast the chilis for 15 minutes until charred around edges.
4. Place them in a bowl then cover with plastic sheet.
5. Let it rest for 15 minutes then peel off the loosed skin.
6. Toss the peeled chilies into the food processor.
7. Then add rest of the ingredients to the chilies then pulse them until smooth.
8. Whisk in water if the paste is too thick.
9. Serve or preserve for later use.

Creamy Lemon Dip
Prep + Cook time: 5 minutes | Serves:4

Nutritional Info (per serving)

Calories	*Fat (g)*	*Protein (g)*	*Carbs (g)*	*Fiber (g)*
17	1	0.9	6.8	0.3

Ingredients:

1 cup paleo mayonnaise	1/2 cup fresh parsley

2-4 tbs. lemon juice to taste

2-4 large cloves garlic to taste

2 tbs. fresh dill

1 teaspoon lemon zest

1/2 teaspoon sea salt

fresh cracked pepper to taste

Directions:

1. Toss everything into the blender.
2. Pulse them well until smooth.
3. Serve fresh.

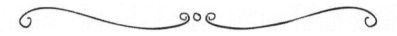

Vegan Basil Pesto

Prep + Cook time: 5 minutes | Serves: 12

Nutritional Info (per serving)

Calories	Fat (g)	Protein (g)	Carbs (g)	Fiber (g)
14	0	0.4	4.1	0.4

Ingredients:

4 cups fresh organic basil

1/2 cup organic walnuts

1/4 cup nutritional yeast

1/4 cup organic extra-virgin olive oil

2 tbs. organic lemon juice

1/2 teaspoon Himalayan pink salt

1/4 teaspoon organic ground black pepper

Directions:

1. Toss everything into a blender.

2. Pulse them well until smooth.
3. Serve fresh.

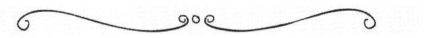

Vegan Cilantro Pesto
Prep + Cook time: 5 minutes | Serves: 12

Nutritional Info (per serving)

Calories	*Fat (g)*	*Protein (g)*	*Carbs (g)*	*Fiber (g)*
20	1.3	0.3	8.5	0.3

Ingredients:

2 cups organic fresh cilantro

1/2 cup organic pine nuts

1/2 cup organic extra-virgin olive oil

1/3 cup nutritional yeast

3 cloves organic garlic

3 tbs. apple cider vinegar

1/2 teaspoon Himalayan pink salt

1/2 teaspoon organic ground black pepper

Directions:

1. Toss everything into the blender.
2. Pulse them well until smooth.
3. Serve fresh.

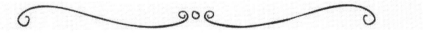

Tomatillo Jalapeno Dip
Prep + Cook time: 5 minutes | Serves: 12

Nutritional Info (per serving)

Calories	Fat (g)	Protein (g)	Carbs (g)	Fiber (g)
19	0.4	0.4	4.8	1.4

Ingredients

3 tomatillos, chopped

1/2 organic onion

1/4 cup organic cilantro

1/8 cup organic lime juice

1/4 cup organic olive oil

1 tbs. apple cider vinegar

1/2 organic jalapeno

1 organic garlic

Pink salt, to taste

Directions:

1. Toss everything into the blender.
2. Pulse them well until smooth.
3. Serve fresh.

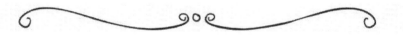

Cauliflower Artichoke Hummus
Prep + Cook time: 45 minutes | Serves: 12

Nutritional Info (per serving)

Calories	Fat (g)	Protein (g)	Carbs (g)	Fiber (g)
8	1.5	0	6.4	2.6

Ingredients:

1 big head cauliflower, florets, washed and dried

Few garlic cloves, unpeeled

3-4 tbs. nutritional yeast

1 tbs. avocado oil

Salt & pepper

1, 9oz jar marinated artichokes, drained and pat dried

11/2 cup extra virgin olive oil

fresh lemon juice, to taste

salt and pepper, to taste

1/4 teaspoon mustard powder

2 tbs. tahini

3 roasted garlic cloves

Directions:

1. Let your oven preheat at 375 degrees F.
2. Toss cauliflower with avocado oil, salt, pepper and yeast in a baking sheet.
3. Place garlic cloves in between the florets.
4. Roast them for 40 minutes then transfer them to a processor.
5. Add drained artichokes and pulse them together until pureed.
6. Pour in some water if it is too thick.
7. Mix well and serve.

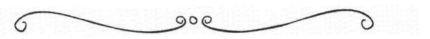

Sweet Potato Hummus

Prep + Cook time: 45 minutes | Serves: 12

Nutritional Info (per serving)

Calories	Fat (g)	Protein (g)	Carbs (g)	Fiber (g)
21	1.2	0.9	17.5	0.3

Ingredients:

1 big sweet potato, whole, washed and dried

4-6 whole garlic cloves, unpeeled

1 teaspoon ghee / avocado oil

1 heaping tbs. tahini

juice of 1/2 lime

1 teaspoon olive oil

sea salt

raw vegetable sticks (for serving)

Directions:

1. Let your oven to preheat at 375 degrees F.
2. Score the sweet potatoes with a fork to poke some holes.
3. Toss these potatoes and garlic with avocado oil.
4. Place them in a baking sheet and bake them for 25 minutes.
5. Remove the garlic and bake the potato more for 15 minutes.
6. Blend the bake veggies with the remaining ingredients until smooth.
7. Serve.

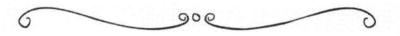

Avocado Hummus

Prep + Cook time: 5 minutes | Serves: 12

Nutritional Info (per serving)

Calories	Fat (g)	Protein (g)	Carbs (g)	Fiber (g)
15	1.1	0.9	4.1	0.3

Ingredients:

2 cup canned chickpeas

2 ripe avocados, cored and peeled

1/3 cup tahini

1/4 cup lime juice

2 cloves garlic

3 tbs. olive oil

1/4 teaspoon cumin

kosher salt

1 tbs. Chopped cilantro, for garnish

Directions:

1. Toss everything into the blender.
2. Pulse them well until smooth.
3. Serve fresh.

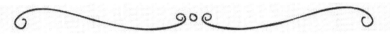

Kale Artichoke Dip

Prep + Cook time: 5 minutes | Serves: 12

Nutritional Info (per serving)

Calories	Fat (g)	Protein (g)	Carbs (g)	Fiber (g)
14	0.1	0.3	4.1	0.1

Ingredients:

1 1/2 cup finely chopped kale

1 tbs. olive oil

Juice of 1/2 lemon

kosher salt

Freshly ground pepper

2 cup Greek yogurt

1/4 cup lectin free mayonnaise

1 tbs. honey

3 green onions, finely chopped

1/3 cup finely chopped red pepper

1/2 carrot, grated

2 garlic cloves, minced

1 1/2 cup finely chopped artichoke hearts

Pita chips, for serving

273

Directions:

1. Toss everything into a suitably sized bowl.
2. Mix well them well until smooth.
3. Serve fresh.

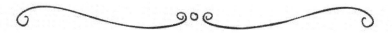

Yogurt Onion Dip
Prep + Cook time: 35 minutes | Serves: 12

Nutritional Info (per serving)

Calories	Fat (g)	Protein (g)	Carbs (g)	Fiber (g)
11	0	2.1	2.6	0.6

Ingredients:

2 onions, thinly sliced

2 tbs. olive oil

2 teaspoon fresh thyme leaves

kosher salt

Freshly ground pepper

1 tbs. apple cider vinegar

2 cups Greek yogurt

Carrot sticks, for serving

Crackers, for serving

Directions:

1. Sauté onion with thyme in a greased pan for 20 minutes until caramelized.
2. Stir in vinegar and cook for a minute then turn off the heat.
3. Combine this onions mixture with the remaining ingredients in a bowl.

4. Allow it to cool then serve.

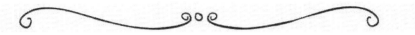

Avocado Lime Dip
Prep + Cook time: 5 minutes | Serves: 8

Nutritional Info (per serving)

Calories	*Fat (g)*	*Protein (g)*	*Carbs (g)*	*Fiber (g)*
15	1.1	0.9	1.4	0.3

Ingredients:

2 ripe avocados

2 cloves garlic, minced

1/2 cup plain Greek yogurt

2 taablespoon lime juice

Kosher salt

Freshly ground black pepper

Pita or tortilla chips and vegetable sticks, for serving

Directions:

1. Toss everything into the blender.
2. Pulse them well until smooth.
3. Serve fresh.

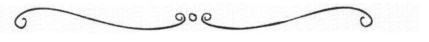

Queso Dip
Prep + Cook time: 5 minutes | Serves: 12

Nutritional Info (per serving)

Calories	*Fat (g)*	*Protein (g)*	*Carbs (g)*	*Fiber (g)*

| 19 | 2.1 | 0.9 | 3.1 | 0.3 |

Ingredients:

2 tbs. almond butter	1 teaspoon chili powder
3 cloves garlic, minced	1/2 teaspoon cumin
1 jalapeno, seeded and diced	Kosher salt and black pepper, to taste
2 tbs. almond flour	1/4 cup plain Greek yogurt
2 cups Silk Unsweetened Coconut Milk	1 avocado, halved, seeded, peeled and diced
3 cups shredded parmesan cheese	2 tbs. chopped fresh cilantro leaves

Directions:

1. Mash avocados in a suitablysized bowl using a fork.
2. Fold in the remainingingredients and mix well.
3. Enjoy or preserve for later use.

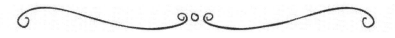

French Onion Dip
Prep + Cook time: 35 minutes | Serves: 12

Nutritional Info (per serving)

Calories	*Fat (g)*	*Protein (g)*	*Carbs (g)*	*Fiber (g)*
17	1.1	0.9	2.1	0.3

Ingredients:

2 tbs. olive oil

3 medium onions, peeled and diced

2 cloves garlic, minced

1 1/2 cups low-fat Greek yogurt

2 teaspoons Worcestershire sauce, to taste

1 teaspoon salt

1/2 teaspoon black pepper

pinch of cayenne

Directions:

1. Add butter to a stockpot and heat it.
2. Stir in onions and sauté them for 30 minutes until caramelized.
3. Add garlic and sauté for 2 minutes then turn off the heat.
4. Allow the mixture to cool then transfer to a blender jug.
5. Toss in the remaining ingredients and pulse them together until smooth.
6. Serve and preserve for later use.

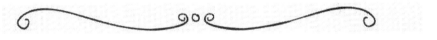

Pumpkin Dip

Prep + Cook time: 5 minutes | Serves: 12

Nutritional Info (per serving)

Calories	Fat (g)	Protein (g)	Carbs (g)	Fiber (g)
18	1.1	1.1	2.1	0.5

Ingredients:

1 (8-oz) package light cream cheese

¾ cup canned pureed pumpkin

2 tbs. fat-free vanilla Greek yogurt

¾ teaspoon cinnamon

¼ teaspoon nutmeg

⅛ teaspoon cloves

1½ tbs. Truvia sweetener

½ teaspoon vanilla extract

Nella Wafers and Gingersnaps for dipping

Directions:

1. Toss everything into the blender.
2. Pulse them well until smooth.
3. Serve fresh.

Taco Salsa Dip

Prep + Cook time: 5 minutes | Serves: 12

Nutritional Info (per serving)

Calories	*Fat (g)*	*Protein (g)*	*Carbs (g)*	*Fiber (g)*
15	0.1	0.2	4.1	1.3

Ingredients:

1 cup salsa (mild, medium, or hot)

3/4 cup Greek yogurt

2 to 3 teaspoons taco seasoning

1 cup packed cilantro leaves

Directions:

1. Toss everything into the blender.
2. Pulse them well until smooth.

3. Serve fresh.

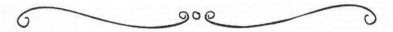

Green Chili Spread

Prep + Cook time: 10 minutes | Serves: 8

Nutritional Info (per serving)

Calories	*Fat (g)*	*Protein (g)*	*Carbs (g)*	*Fiber (g)*
21	1.2	0.2	4.1	1.2

Ingredients:

2 (8 ounce) packages cream cheese, softened

1 cup lectin free mayonnaise

1 (4 ounces) can green chilies, chopped, drained

1 cup grated Parmesan cheese

Directions:

1. Mix mayonnaise with cream cheese in a microwave proof bowl.
2. Fold in jalapeno and green chili.
3. Drizzle cheese on top and heat for 3 minutes in the microwave.
4. Allow it to cool then serve to use.

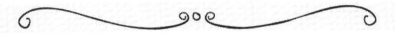

Pumpkin Spice Dip

Prep + Cook time: 5 minutes | Serves: 12

Nutritional Info (per serving)

Calories	Fat (g)	Protein (g)	Carbs (g)	Fiber (g)
20	0.7	0.5	3.4	0.1

Ingredients:

1 cup frozen coconut cream, thawed

1 (5 ounces) package instant vanilla pudding mix

1 (15 ounces) can solid pack pumpkin, diced

1 teaspoon pumpkin pie spice

Directions:

1. Toss everything into the blender.
2. Pulse them well until smooth.
3. Serve fresh.

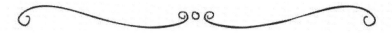

Chicago Spinach Dip

Prep + Cook time: 5 minutes | Serves: 12

Nutritional Info (per serving)

Calories	Fat (g)	Protein (g)	Carbs (g)	Fiber (g)
17	1.2	0.9	2.4	0.4

Ingredients:

1 (10 ounces) package frozen spinach, thawed and drained

1 cup sour cream

1 cup lectin free mayonnaise

3/4 cup chopped green onions

2 teaspoons dried parsley

1 teaspoon lemon juice   1/2 teaspoon seasoned salt

Directions:

1. Toss everything into a suitablysized bowl.
2. Mix them well until smooth.
3. Serve fresh.

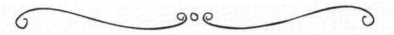

Roasted Red Pepper Dip
Prep + Cook time: 35 minutes | Serves: 12

Nutritional Info (per serving)

Calories	*Fat (g)*	*Protein (g)*	*Carbs (g)*	*Fiber (g)*
21	1.1	0.8	3.4	1.6

Ingredients:

1 cup roasted red peppers, peeled, deseeded and diced

3/4-pound shredded parmesan cheese

1 (8 ounces) package cream cheese, softened

1 cup lectin free mayonnaise

1 tbs. minced onion

1 clove garlic, minced

2 tbs. prepared Dijon-style mustard

Directions:

1. Let your oven preheat at 350 degrees F.
2. Toss everything together in a baking pan.
3. Bake it for 20 minutes until it bubbles.
4. Serve.

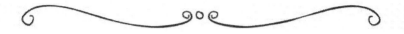

Red Chili Sauce

Prep + Cook time: 10 minutes | Serves: 8

Nutritional Info (per serving)

Calories	*Fat (g)*	*Protein (g)*	*Carbs (g)*	*Fiber (g)*
24	0.5	1.5	8.4	2.1

Ingredients:

3 dried Ancho

Water

1 large clove garlic

2 whole cloves, crushed

2 black peppercorns, crushed

1/2 teaspoon of salt, more to taste

Olive oil

Directions:

1. Deseed the sliced chili and roast them in a dry skillet for 1 minute.
2. Toss everything into the blender.
3. Pulse them well until smooth.
4. Serve fresh.

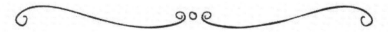

Snacks and Appetizer Recipes

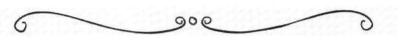

Avocado Taco Cups
Prep + Cook time: 35 minutes | Serves: 4

Nutritional Info (per serving)

Calories	*Fat (g)*	*Protein (g)*	*Carbs (g)*	*Fiber (g)*
227	0.5	0.8	23	0.3

Ingredients:

Taco Cups

Avocado oil for greasing

1 cup cassava flour

1/2 cup unsweetened coconut milk

1/4 cup almond butter

1/4 cup warm water

Avocado filling:

1 tbs. avocado oil

1/2 medium onion finely chopped

2 teaspoons chili powder

2 teaspoons ground cumin

1 teaspoon coriander

1 teaspoon coconut aminos

1/2 teaspoon dried oregano

1/2 teaspoon paprika

1/4 teaspoon garlic powder

2 avocadoes, peeled, pitted and mashed

sea salt and black pepper, to taste

hot sauce, shredded lettuce,

Directions:

1. Let your oven preheat at 425 degrees F. Grease a muffin tray with avocado oil.
2. Mix all the taco cups ingredients in a mixer to form a dough.

3. Divide the dough into each greased muffin cup. Press it firmly.
4. Bake the crust for 20 minutes in the preheated oven.
5. Meanwhile, mix avocado filling ingredients in a bowl.
6. Divide the filling into the baked taco cups.
7. Serve fresh.

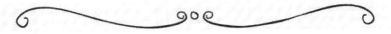

Rainbow Fries

Prep + Cook time: 35 minutes | Serves: 4

Nutritional Info (per serving)

Calories	*Fat (g)*	*Protein (g)*	*Carbs (g)*	*Fiber (g)*
117	12.5	1.9g	29.4g	4.2g

Ingredients:

4 purple carrots, peeled, halved, and cut lengthwise

2 yuca roots, peeled, and cut into thick strips

2 sweet potatoes, peeled and slicedinto thick strips

3 tbs. extra-virgin olive oil

2 teaspoons granulated garlic

2 teaspoons sea salt

black pepper

3 tbs. grainy mustard

Directions:

1. Let your oven preheat at 450 degrees F.
2. Toss the sliced veggies with salt, pepper, garlic, and olive oil.
3. Spread them in two baking sheets.

4. Bake them for 20 minutes until crispy.
5. Serve warm.

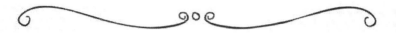

Swiss Chard Fritters

Prep + Cook time: 15 minutes | Serves: 4

Nutritional Info (per serving)

Calories	Fat (g)	Protein (g)	Carbs (g)	Fiber (g)
156	14.2	11.6g	31.5g	1.1g

Ingredients:

1 bunch of Swiss chard, torn

3 cloves garlic, chopped

1/2 teaspoon ground cumin

sea salt and black pepper

2 ounces crumbled goat cheese

1/2 cup cassava flour

4 tbs. extra-virgin olive oil, divided

organic sour cream for serving

Directions:

1. Add Swiss chard, salt, pepper, garlic, and cumin to a food processor.
2. Finely chop this mixture in the processor.
3. Mix this chard mixture with flour, and cheese.
4. Make ¼ inch thick patties out of this mixture.
5. Sear the patties for 4 minutes per side in the heated olive oil in a pan.

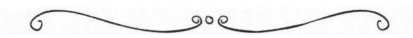

6. Serve.

Ravioli Wraps

Prep + Cook time: 15 minutes | Serves: 4

Nutritional Info (per serving)

Calories	*Fat (g)*	*Protein (g)*	*Carbs (g)*	*Fiber (g)*
311	15.5	2.9g	41.6g	2.4g

Ingredients:

RAVIOLI

4 tbs. olive oil divided

1 10-oz package frozen, spinach chopped and thawed

1/4 cup imported Italian mascarpone

1/4 cup grated Parmigiano-Reggiano

5 square coconut wraps

2 large pastured eggs whisked with 1 teaspoon water

BASIL PESTO

2 cups packed fresh basil leaves

1/4 cup pine nuts

1-ounce Parmigiano-Reggiano crumbled

2 cloves garlic

1/2 cup olive oil

Directions:

1. Sauté spinach for 2 minutes in 2 tbs. olive oil in a skillet.
2. Mix the spinach with Parmigiano and mascarpone in a bowl.
3. Place 2.5 wraps on a board in a line and brush them with egg wash.
4. Add dollops of prepared spinach are filling in the four corners of the wraps.
5. Separate the four corners by cutting them with a ravioli cutter.
6. Blend the basil pesto ingredients in a blender until smooth.
7. Add 2 tbsp oil in a saucepan and heat it.
8. Sear the ravioli for 3 minutes in two batches.
9. Serve with prepared pesto.
10. Enjoy.

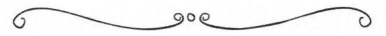

Onion Rings
Prep + Cook time: 25 minutes | Serves: 2

Nutritional Info (per serving)

Calories	*Fat (g)*	*Protein (g)*	*Carbs (g)*	*Fiber (g)*
247	18.5	3.6g	21.6g	2.2g

Ingredients:

2 cups cassava flour

1 tbs. chili powder

1 teaspoon baking soda

1 1/4 cups club soda, chilled

1 medium onion, thickly sliced and separate in rings

1/4 teaspoon salt

1/4 teaspoon garlic powder

1/4 teaspoon black pepper

Directions:

1. Combine all the ingredients except onion, to prepare the batter.
2. Dip the onion rings in this batter to coat well.
3. Shake off the excess and place each ring in a greased baking sheet.
4. Bake the rings at 425 degrees F in the preheated oven until golden brown.
5. Serve warm.

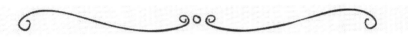

Prosciutto Wrapped Artichoke Hearts
Prep + Cook time: 5 minutes | Serves: 1

Nutritional Info (per serving)

Calories	*Fat (g)*	*Protein (g)*	*Carbs (g)*	*Fiber (g)*
169	11.5	15.8	10.4	3.5

Ingredients:

1 jar artichokes hearts, drained and pat dried

5 slices of Prosciutto di Parma

1 garlic clove, whole, minced

6 mushroom chunks

2 fresh thyme stems

a small handful of grated Parmigiano Reggiano

avocado oil for cooking

dry oregano

Directions:

1. Let your oven preheat at 450 degrees F. Layer a baking sheet with wax paper.

2. Drain the artichoke hearts and drain each heart with one prosciutto slice
3. Place the wrapped hearts in the baking sheet along with mushrooms.
4. Top the wraps with avocado oil and thyme.
5. Bake these stuffed wraps for 15 mins in the preheated oven.
6. Drizzle Reggiano and oregano on top.
7. Enjoy.

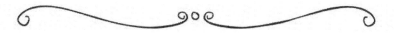

Strawberry Salsa

Prep + Cook time: 15 minutes | Serves: 2

Nutritional Info (per serving)

Calories	Fat (g)	Protein (g)	Carbs (g)	Fiber (g)
144	3.5	1.9	8.4	0.1

Ingredients:

4 big strawberries, chopped

3 tbsp red onion, finely chopped

a handful of fresh chopped cilantro

1/2 lime, juice

Salt, to taste

Pepper, to taste

2 tbsp olive oil

Directions:

1. Put everything into a large bowl.
2. Mix well.
3. Serve fresh.

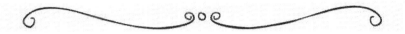

Baked Artichokes with Hazelnuts Pesto

Prep + Cook time: 40 minutes | Serves: 2

Nutritional Info (per serving)

Calories	*Fat (g)*	*Protein (g)*	*Carbs (g)*	*Fiber (g)*
196	0.5	0.9g	32.5g	2.1g

Ingredients:

For pesto:

1/2 cup hazelnuts

2 tbsp nutritional yeast

1/2 cup pitted green olives

bunch of parsley

4 tbsp extra virgin olive oil

The artichoke:

1 big whole artichoke, cut in half

one lemon (for juice)

2 tbsp extra virgin olive oil

garlic powder

Directions:

1. Add all the pesto ingredients to the food processor.
2. Blend it until it forms a coarse mixture.
3. Place the sliced artichokes in the baking sheet.
4. Top the artichokes with this prepared pesto.
5. Drizzle lemon juice, olive oil, and garlic powder on top.
6. Bake them for 30 minutes.
7. Serve warm.

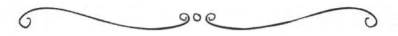

Parmigiano Reggiano Chips

Prep + Cook time: 15 minutes | Serves: 4

Nutritional Info (per serving)

Calories	Fat (g)	Protein (g)	Carbs (g)	Fiber (g)
110	21.5	0.3	0.4	0

Ingredients:

1 packed cup freshly grated Parmigiano Reggiano

Black pepper to taste

Salt, to taste

Directions:

1. Let your oven preheat at 400 degrees F for baking.
2. Layer a baking tray with parchment sheet and keep it aside.
3. Grate the Reggiano and spread the grated cheese over the baking parchment paper.
4. Bake it for 9 minutes until crispy and golden.
5. Break the cheese bake into small chips.
6. Drizzle salt and pepper on top.
7. Enjoy.

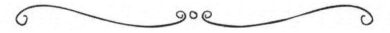

Curried Sardines in Radicchio Cups

Prep + Cook time: 15 minutes | Serves: 6

Nutritional Info (per serving)

Calories	Fat (g)	Protein (g)	Carbs (g)	Fiber (g)

Ingredients:

2 cans sardines

Curry Mayo Sauce:

3/4 cup avocado mayo

2 tbsp finely chopped pear or apple

2 tbsp capers, rinsed and pat dried

For Serving:

6 radicchios, washed, dried and cut in half

6 slices of watermelon radish

1 or 2 hard-boiled egg (pasture raised), each cut in 6 pieces

2 tbsp finely chopped red onion

1 tsp curry powder

1/2 tsp Turmeric Tonic powder

1 heaping tbsp goat yogurt

Parsley, chopped

extra virgin olive oil

pepper

Directions:

1. Mash the drained sardines in a bowl then whisk in sauce ingredients.
2. Place the radicchio boats in the serving plates.
3. Divide Sardines mixture in the boats.
4. Top the filling with sliced boiled eggs, radish, pepper and parsley.
5. Drizzle olive oil on top.
6. Enjoy.

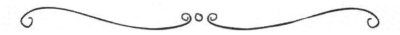

Italian Meatballs

Prep + Cook time: 35 minutes | Serves: 6

Nutritional Info (per serving)

Calories	*Fat (g)*	*Protein (g)*	*Carbs (g)*	*Fiber (g)*
306	12.5	15.9g	4.4g	0.5g

Ingredients:

1 lb 100% ground grass-fed beef

1 big red onion

2 big garlic cloves

1 big bunch flat leaf parsley

1 bunch fresh basil leaves

5 medium button mushrooms

2 pasture raised eggs

1 tbsp cassava flour for the mixture, more for coating of meatballs

spices: dry oregano, salt (about 1 tsp) and pepper

Directions:

1. Let your oven preheat at 375 degrees F.
2. Finely chop mushrooms, garlic, onion, basil and parsley in a food processor.
3. Mix the chopped veggies with beef, eggs, spices, salt and flour in a bowl.
4. Make small meatballs out of this mixture.
5. Place these balls in a baking sheet.
6. Bake these balls for 20 minutes or more until brown.
7. Serve warm.

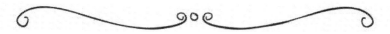

Chicken Pot Pie

Prep + Cook time: 35 minutes | Serves: 4

Nutritional Info (per serving)

Calories	*Fat (g)*	*Protein (g)*	*Carbs (g)*	*Fiber (g)*
215	14.5	10.9g	6.4g	0.1g

Ingredients:

CRUST:

1 cup almond flour

1/2 cup coconut flour

1/2 cup tapioca starch

1/2 cup almond butter

1/2 teaspoon fine sea salt

1 whole pastured egg + 1 egg white (egg wash)

FILLING:

2 cups of cooked chicken, chopped

2 tbs. avocado oil

1 sweet (or yellow) onion, diced

1 medium carrot, peeled and diced

2 cups mushrooms, chopped

1 bunch fresh parsley

1/2 bunch asparagus, chopped

1 cup chicken broth

1/4 cup organic coconut cream

salt and pepper to taste

2 tbsp arrowroot powder

Directions:

1. Let your oven preheat at 375 degrees F.

2. Mix all the ingredients for crust in a bowl to form the dough.
3. Wrap this dough in a plastic sheet then refrigerate for 30 minutes.
4. Sauté mushrooms and carrots in the avocado oil in a pan for 10 minutes.
5. Stir in all the remaining ingredients for the fillings.
6. Cook this mixture for 5 minutes.
7. Remove the dough from the refrigerate and divide it into two halves.
8. Take one half and divide it into greased molds.
9. Press the dough against the base.
10. Divide the prepared fillings in the molds.
11. Take the remaining half of reserved dough and divide it into equal sized pieces
12. Spread the dough into mold sized circles.
13. Cover each mold and bake them for 20 minutes.
14. Serve.

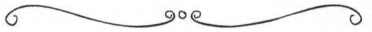

Avocado Nori Rolls
Prep + Cook time: 15 minutes | Serves: 4

Nutritional Info (per serving)

Calories	*Fat (g)*	*Protein (g)*	*Carbs (g)*	*Fiber (g)*
114	1.5	16	1.4	0.2

Ingredients:

4-5 oz. wild caught salmon fillet, cooked and flaked

1/2 big avocado, sliced

3 oz. almond cream cheese

1/2 cup pitted kalamata olives, drained

4 roasted nori sheets

Directions:

1. Spread the nori sheets and layer them with cream cheese.
2. Place the salmon, avocado, and olives on top.
3. Roll the sheets into tightly packed rolls.
4. Serve.

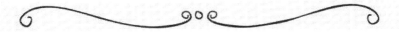

Sushi Rolls with Cauliflower Rice

Prep + Cook time: 25 minutes | Serves: 3

Nutritional Info (per serving)

Calories	Fat (g)	Protein (g)	Carbs (g)	Fiber (g)
127	4.2	7.1	13.4	1

Ingredients:

For Cauliflower Rice:

1 medium cauliflower head, riced

1 tbsp avocado oil

2 tsp coconut aminos

1 tbsp rice vinegar

1 tsp salt

For Filling:

4 thick strips of green mango

1/2 avocado cut in long stripes

1 cup (or less) of cooked crab meat

2, 3 medium cooked wild caught shrimps cut in long stripes

3 sheets roasted Nori

few tbsp Avocado mayonnaise

FOR SERVING:

Wasabi paste

pickled ginger

2, 3 red radishes thinly sliced

coconut aminos

Directions:

1. Sauté cauliflower rice for 3 minutes in avocado oil in a pan.
2. Stir in vinegar, salt, and aminos.
3. Transfer the rice to a separate bowl and allow it to cool.
4. Spread the nori sheet on the bamboo sheet and spread the cauliflower rice over it.
5. Place all the fillings at the center of the nori.
6. Roll them into sushi and then serve with wasabi, radish, and ginger.

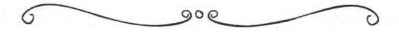

Citrus and Aniseeds Olives
Prep + Cook time: 15 minutes | Serves: 4

Nutritional Info (per serving)

Calories	Fat (g)	Protein (g)	Carbs (g)	Fiber (g)
91	3.5	1.9	0.4	0.3

Ingredients

1 cup pitted olives, drained, rinsed and pat dried

3 tbsps olive oil

zest of 1-2 organic lemons

zest of 1 organic orange

1/4 tsp coriander powder

1/4 tsp fennel seeds

1/4 tsp aniseeds

Directions:

1. Add oil to a small pan and toss in olives.
2. Stir in all the remaining ingredients.
3. Sauté them for 5 minutes.
4. Serve.

Mushrooms Stuffed with Almond Ricotta

Prep + Cook time: 35 minutes | Serves: 10

Nutritional Info (per serving)

Calories	Fat (g)	Protein (g)	Carbs (g)	Fiber (g)
107	7.5	3.4	22.6	0.2

Ingredients:

10 mini Portobello mushrooms

1/2 cup almond ricotta

1 tbsp extra virgin olive oil

2 tbsp fresh oregano leaves, chopped

1 garlic clove, finely chopped

Avocado oil

salt and pepper

Directions:

1. Let your oven preheat at 400 degrees F.
2. Clean and destem the mushrooms then pat them dry.
3. Mix the remaining ingredients and stuff the mushrooms with this mixture.
4. Place the mushrooms in the baking sheet.

5. Bake them for 30 minutes until well cooked.
6. Serve warm.

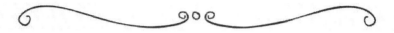

Almond Bread Bites

Prep + Cook time: 45 minutes | Serves: 4

Nutritional Info (per serving)

Calories	*Fat (g)*	*Protein (g)*	*Carbs (g)*	*Fiber (g)*
177	12.5	0.6g	14	0.2g

Ingredients

1/2 cup full-fat coconut milk

1 1/2 cup cassava flour

1/2 cup avocado oil

2 pasture raised eggs

1 cup almond

2 cups Pecorino Romano cheese

Directions:

1. Let your oven preheat at 410 degrees F.
2. Grease a muffin tray with some oil and keep it aside.
3. Whisk eggs with coconut milk and avocado oil in a large bowl.
4. Toss in the remaining ingredients and mix well to make a smooth dough.
5. Make 12 balls out of this dough and place one ball in each muffin cup.
6. Place 1 to 2 almonds on top of each muffin cup.
7. Bake them for 30 minutes.
8. Serve.

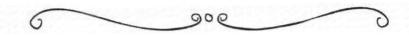

Cranberries Almond Crackers

Prep + Cook time: 25 minutes | Serves: 4

Nutritional Info (per serving)

Calories	Fat (g)	Protein (g)	Carbs (g)	Fiber (g)
154	4.5	3.8	13	2.1

Ingredients:

1 cup blanched almond flour

1 tbsp flax meal

4 tbsp unsweetened dry cranberries

2 tbsp hemp seeds

1 spring fresh rosemary leaves

2 tsp extra virgin olive oil

2 tbsp cold water

pinch of salt

Directions:

1. Let your oven preheat at 350 degrees F.
2. Put everything for crackers in the food processor except the hemp seeds.
3. Grind the mixture in the processor until crumbly.
4. Fold in the hemp seeds and pulse for 5 seconds.
5. Spread the mixture in a baking sheet with parchment paper.
6. Slice the sheet using a pizza cutter into small chunks.
7. Bake them in the oven until golden brown.
8. Serve.

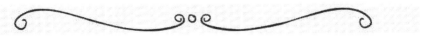

Spicy Sweet Potato Snack

Prep + Cook time: 25 minutes | Serves: 2

Nutritional Info (per serving)

Calories	Fat (g)	Protein (g)	Carbs (g)	Fiber (g)
241	0.2	0.4g	33.4g	0g

Ingredients:

2 sweet potatoes, peeled and cubed

Dry spice mix: sage, thyme, yellow mustard, black pepper, coarse salt

1 tsp arrowroot powder

Avocado oil

Directions:

1. Let your oven preheat at 375 degrees F.
2. Toss the sweet potatoes with avocado oil, arrowroot powder, and spices.
3. Bake them for 10 minutes until al dente.
4. Serve warm.

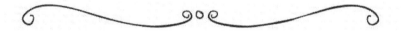

Chicken Salad Nori Rolls with Organic Miracle Rice

Prep + Cook time: 5 minutes | Serves: 1

Nutritional Info (per serving)

Calories	Fat (g)	Protein (g)	Carbs (g)	Fiber (g)
152	1.2	2	14	1.3

Ingredients:

FOR THE ROLLS:

1 pack Organic Miracle
Rice, cooked

3 roasted Nori sheets

1 cup of homemade chicken
salad

few handfuls of baby
arugula

FOR SERVING:

red radishes, finely sliced

pickled ginger

wasabi paste

Hot sauce

Coconut aminos

Directions:

1. Spread a nori sheet on a bamboo sheet.
2. Evenly spread a thin layer of cooked rice over the nori
   sheets.
3. Place the chicken salad and arugula at the center of the
   nori sheet.
4. Start rolling the nori sheet to make a sushi roll.
5. Repeat the same process with the rest of the nori sheets.
6. Serve fresh with the serving ingredients.
7. Enjoy.

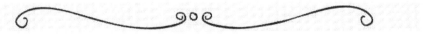

Gingerbread in a Mug
Prep + Cook time: 10 minutes | Serves: 1

Nutritional Info (per serving)

Calories	Fat (g)	Protein (g)	Carbs (g)	Fiber (g)
227	0.5	0.4	24.7	0.1

Ingredients:

1 tbs. almond butter, softened

1 tbs. coconut flour

1 tbs. tigernut or cassava flour

1/2 teaspoon ground ginger

1/4 teaspoon cinnamon

pinch each of allspice, cloves, and nutmeg

1/2 teaspoon baking powder

2 teaspoons maple-flavored erythritol syrup

1/2 teaspoon apple cider vinegar

1/2 tbs. water

1 egg, lightly beaten

Directions:

1. Whisk egg, cider, and syrup in a bowl.
2. Stir in all the remaining ingredients.
3. Mix well then pour the batter into a mug.
4. Bake this batter in the microwave for 1.5 minutes at high temperature.
5. Serve warm with cinnamon and butter on top.

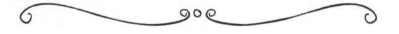

Oven-Baked Okra Bites
Prep + Cook time: 35 minutes | Serves: 4

Nutritional Info (per serving)

Calories	Fat (g)	Protein (g)	Carbs (g)	Fiber (g)

Ingredients:

For the okra:

12 organic okra pods (sliced)

2 tbs. 100% pure avocado oil

For the bread crumbs:

1/4 cup almond flour

1/4 cup nutritional yeast

1/4 teaspoon organic
ground garlic powder

1/4 teaspoon organic
ground cayenne pepper

1/4 teaspoon Himalayan
pink salt

Directions:

1. Let your oven preheat at 425 degrees F.
2. Toss all the ingredients for breadcrumbs in a shallow bowl.
3. Slice okra and rub the pieces with avocado oil.
4. Dredge the okra in the breadcrumbs and coat them well.
5. Place the coated okra in a greased baking sheet.
6. Bake them for 10 minutes then flip all the pieces.
7. Again, bake the pieces for 10 minutes.
8. Enjoy warm.

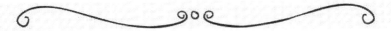

Pumpkin Spice Crackers with Sea Salt
Prep + Cook time: 25 minutes | Serves: 4

Nutritional Info (per serving)

Calories	Fat (g)	Protein (g)	Carbs (g)	Fiber (g)
143	0.3	0.4	22.7	0.2

Ingredients

Crackers:

2 cups almond flour

1 tbs. avocado oil

1 flax egg (3 tbs. water mixed with 1 tbs. ground flax)

2 teaspoons organic pumpkin spice

1/2 teaspoon Himalayan pink salt

1/4 teaspoon black pepper

1/8 teaspoon garlic powder

Topping:

Sea Salt

Directions:

1. Let your oven preheat at 350 degrees F.
2. Mix the flax seeds with water in a large bowl.
3. Toss in the remaining ingredients for crackers.
4. Mix well then spread this mixture in a baking sheet lined with wax paper.
5. Drizzle sea salt on top then bake it for 15 minutes until golden.
6. Break the baked sheet into pieces.
7. Serve.

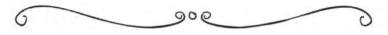

Cheesy Garlic Breadsticks
Prep + Cook time: 5 minutes | Serves: 1

Nutritional Info (per serving)

Calories	*Fat (g)*	*Protein (g)*	*Carbs (g)*	*Fiber (g)*
153	12.3	9	27.1	1.1

Ingredients:

For the breadsticks:

2 cups almond flour

2 cups Daiya Mozzarella Cheese

1 teaspoon organic extra-virgin olive oil

1 teaspoon organic ground garlic powder

1/2 teaspoon Himalayan pink salt

3 flax eggs (3 tbs. flax seeds ground + 9 tbs. purified water)

For the garlic topping:

4 cloves organic garlic (freshly crushed)

1/8 teaspoon Himalayan pink salt

1 tbs. organic extra-virgin olive oil

1/8 teaspoon organic ground black pepper

1 tbs. organic dried oregano

Directions:

1. Let your oven preheat at 350 degrees F.
2. Combine all the ingredients for the breadsticks in a bowl.
3. Spread this mixture in a baking dish with a parchment sheet.

4. Bake them for 20 minutes in the preheated oven.
5. Meanwhile, combine all the ingredients for toppings.
6. Pour this mixture over the baked breadstick sheet.
7. Once set, slice and serve.
8. Enjoy.

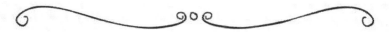

Turmeric Sweet Potato Fries
Prep + Cook time: 25 minutes | Serves: 4

Nutritional Info (per serving)

Calories	Fat (g)	Protein (g)	Carbs (g)	Fiber (g)
143	1.3	2.9	33.2	0.4

Ingredients:

1 large sweet potato, peeled and slice into thick fries

1 tbs. 100% pure avocado oil

For the seasoning:

1/2 teaspoon organic turmeric powder

1/2 teaspoon organic ground black pepper

1/2 teaspoon organic cayenne pepper

1/2 teaspoon Himalayan pink salt

2 tbs. nutritional yeast

Directions:

1. Let your oven preheat at 425 degrees F.
2. Toss the fries with avocado oil in a baking sheet.
3. Mix all the spices and sprinkles them on the potatoes liberally.

4. Toss well to coat and spread them in a baking sheet.
5. Bake them for 20 minutes.
6. Serve warm.

Oven-Baked Fried Artichokes
Prep + Cook time: 25 minutes | Serves: 4

Nutritional Info (per serving)

Calories	*Fat (g)*	*Protein (g)*	*Carbs (g)*	*Fiber (g)*
185	1.5	4.4	16g	0.3g

Ingredients:

For the seasoning:

1/2 cup almond flour

1/2 cup nutritional yeast

1/2 teaspoon organic ground garlic

1/2 teaspoon organic ground cayenne pepper

1/2 teaspoon Himalayan pink salt

For the artichokes:

1 can artichoke hearts (drained)

1 tbs. 100% pure avocado oil

Directions:

1. Let your oven preheat to 425 degrees.
2. Combine all the ingredients for seasoning mixture in a bowl.

3. Place the artichoke pieces in a baking sheet lined with wax paper.
4. Rub the artichoke with avocado oil first then sprinkle the seasonings on top.
5. Bake them for 15 minutes until golden.
6. Enjoy.

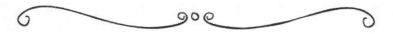

Thyme and Garlic Crackers
Prep + Cook time: 25 minutes | Serves: 4

Nutritional Info (per serving)

Calories	Fat (g)	Protein (g)	Carbs (g)	Fiber (g)
136	0.5	0.3	25.2	0.4

Ingredients:

2 cups almond flour

1 tbs. organic fresh thyme (chopped)

1 tbs. 100% organic pure avocado oil

1/2 teaspoon organic ground garlic powder

1/2 teaspoon organic ground black pepper

1/2 teaspoon Himalayan pink salt

1 flax egg (1 tbs. organic ground flax + 3 tbs. filtered/purified water)

Directions:

1. Let your oven preheat at 350 degrees F.
2. Mix the flax ground with water to make the flax egg and keep it aside.
3. Toss all ingredients for the cracker in a bowl.
4. Stir in flax egg and mix well using a fork.

5. Spread this mixture evenly in a baking sheet lined with wax paper.
6. Bake it for 15 minutes until golden brown from top.
7. Allow them to cool then break into pieces.
8. Enjoy.

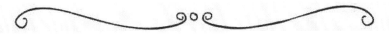

Oven-Baked Avocado Fries
Prep + Cook time: 15 minutes | Serves: 4

Nutritional Info (per serving)

Calories	*Fat (g)*	*Protein (g)*	*Carbs (g)*	*Fiber (g)*
341	8.5	16.9	41.1	3.1

Ingredients:

2 organic avocados, pitted and cut into thick slices

1/2 cup homemade almond milk

For the bread crumbs:

1/2 cup almond flour

1/2 cup nutritional yeast

1/2 teaspoon organic ground garlic powder

1/2 teaspoon organic ground smoked paprika

1/2 teaspoon Himalayan pink salt

Directions:

1. Let your oven preheat at 420 degrees F.
2. Toss all the ingredients for bread crumbs in a shallow bowl.
3. Dip the sliced avocado strips in the milk.
4. Dredge the slices in the bread crumbs mixture.

5. Place them in a greased baking sheet.
6. Bake them for 10 minutes until crispy.
7. Enjoy.

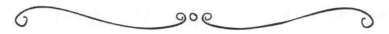

Cheesy Baked Kale Chips
Prep + Cook time: 25 minutes | Serves: 6

Nutritional Info (per serving)

Calories	*Fat (g)*	*Protein (g)*	*Carbs (g)*	*Fiber (g)*
176	8.5	3.5	6.4	2.6

Ingredients:

2 cups organic kale (de-stemmed), torn

1 tbs. 100% pure avocado oil

2 tbs. nutritional yeast

1/2 teaspoon Himalayan pink salt

Directions:

1. Let your oven preheat at 350 degrees F.
2. Toss the kale with all the ingredients in a baking sheet.
3. Bake them for 10 minutes or more until crispy.
4. Serve warm.

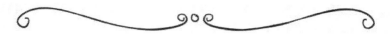

Crispy Zucchini Bites
Prep + Cook time: 35 minutes | Serves: 4

Nutritional Info (per serving)

Calories	*Fat (g)*	*Protein (g)*	*Carbs (g)*	*Fiber (g)*

182	3.6	4.9	24.1	0.7

Ingredients:

Bites:

2 medium zucchinis, thinly sliced

2 tbs. avocado oil

Bread crumbs Mixture:

1/4 teaspoon garlic powder	1/4 cup nutritional yeast
1/4 cup almond flour	1/4 teaspoon salt
1/4 teaspoon cayenne pepper	

Directions:

1. Let your oven preheat at 425 degrees F.
2. Toss all the ingredients for breadcrumbs in a shallow bowl.
3. Slice zucchini and rub the pieces with avocado oil.
4. Dredge the slices in the breadcrumbs and coat them well.
5. Place the coated zucchini slices in a greased baking sheet.
6. Bake them for 10 minutes then flip all the pieces.
7. Again, bake the pieces for 10-15 minutes until crispy.
8. Enjoy warm.

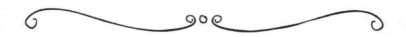

Dessert Recipes

Walnut Fudge

Prep + Cook time: 15 minutes | Serves: 4

Nutritional Info (per serving)

Calories	*Fat (g)*	*Protein (g)*	*Carbs (g)*	*Fiber (g)*
246	3.6	5.8	31.2	1.6

Ingredients:

1 cup organic coconut oil, melted

1/4 cup organic almond butter

1/4 cup organic raw cacao powder

1/4 cup organic walnuts (chopped)

1/4 cup organic date nectar

1 teaspoon organic vanilla bean powder

Directions:

1. Combine all the ingredients for the fudge in a medium-sized bowl until smooth.
2. Transfer the mixture to a 5x9 inch bread pan.
3. Freeze the fudge for 60 minutes until it hardens.
4. Slice and serve.

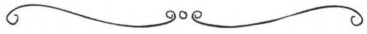

Cacao Pecan Balls

Prep + Cook time: 10 minutes | Serves: 6

Nutritional Info (per serving)

Calories	*Fat (g)*	*Protein (g)*	*Carbs (g)*	*Fiber (g)*

Ingredients:

1 cup organic raw pecans, chopped

1/2 cup organic almond butter

1/4 cup almond flour

1/4 cup organic raw cacao powder

2 tbs. organic hemp oil

2 tbs. organic maca powder

1 tbs. organic date nectar

1/2 teaspoon organic vanilla bean powder

Directions:

1. Toss all the ingredients to a processor until it forms a thick paste.
2. Make small balls using a spoon and place them cover a baking sheet.
3. Refrigerate it for 30 minutes.
4. Serve.

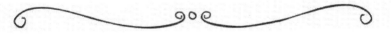

Lemon Meltaway Balls
Prep + Cook time: 10 minutes | Serves: 8

Nutritional Info (per serving)

Calories	*Fat (g)*	*Protein (g)*	*Carbs (g)*	*Fiber (g)*
262	9.9	2.1	18.1	1.3

Ingredients:

1 1/2 cups almond flour

1/4 cup organic lemon juice

1/4 cup organic coconut oil

1/4 cup organic erythritol syrup

1/3 cup organic coconut flour

1 tbs. organic lemon zest

1/2 teaspoon organic pure vanilla extract

1-2 pinches Himalayan pink salt

Directions:

1. Add everything to a processor and pulse until it forms a smooth dough.
2. Make small balls out of this mixture place them on a baking sheet.
3. Refrigerate them for 15 minutes.
4. Roll the balls in coconut oil, then in coconut flakes and sugar.
5. Again, place them in a baking pan lined with wax paper.
6. Refrigerate them for 30 minutes.
7. Enjoy.

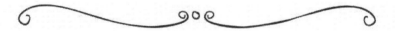

Vanilla Chocolate Pudding
Prep + Cook time: 10 minutes | Serves: 4

Nutritional Info (per serving)

Calories	Fat (g)	Protein (g)	Carbs (g)	Fiber (g)
213	4.5	5	10.8	1.1

Ingredients:

4 organic avocados (pitted)

1/2 cup organic raw coconut nectar

1 teaspoon organic vanilla bean powder

1/4 cup organic raw cacao powder

1 can organic full-fat coconut milk, hard part only

Directions:

1. Put everything into a blender jar.
2. Pulse the ingredients together until smooth.
3. Refrigerate well until chilled.
4. Serve with desired garnish.
5. Enjoy.

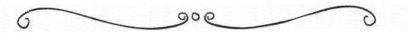

Pistachio Sesame Seed Balls
Prep + Cook time: 10 minutes | Serves: 6

Nutritional Info (per serving)

Calories	*Fat (g)*	*Protein (g)*	*Carbs (g)*	*Fiber (g)*
360	11.3	16.3	26.1	1.4

Ingredients:

1/2 cup organic almond butter

1 cup organic medjool dates (pitted)

1/2 cup organic pistachios

1 tbs. organic coconut oil

1/2 cup organic sesame seeds

Directions:

1. Put everything into a food processor except sesame seeds.
2. Press the button to coarsely chop the mixture.
3. Fold in the sesame seeds and mix well with your hands.
4. Make small balls out of this mixture.
5. Refrigerate them for 30 minutes.
6. Serve and enjoy.

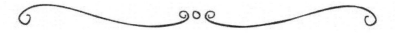

Pecan Pie Truffles

Prep + Cook time: 10 minutes | Serves: 4

Nutritional Info (per serving)

Calories	Fat (g)	Protein (g)	Carbs (g)	Fiber (g)
312	1.4	2.1	14.9	0.4

Ingredients:

1 cup organic pecans

8 organic medjool dates (pitted)

1/2 teaspoon organic vanilla bean powder

Directions:

1. Coarsely grind every ingredienttogether in a food processor.
2. Make small balls out of the well-combined mixture.
3. Refrigerate for 15 minutes.
4. Serve and enjoy.

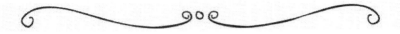

Moringa Ice Cream

Prep + Cook time: 10 minutes | Serves: 4

Nutritional Info (per serving)

Calories	*Fat (g)*	*Protein (g)*	*Carbs (g)*	*Fiber (g)*
296	9.9	10	16.3	0.1

Ingredients

Ice cream:

1 can organic full-fat coconut milk

1/4 - 1/2 cup organic granular sweetener

2 teaspoons organic moringa powder

1 teaspoon organic baobab powder

For the mix-in:

1/2 cup organic raw cacao nibs

Directions:

1. Put everything into the blender jug.
2. Blend them together until smooth.
3. Transfer the mixture to an ice maker and churn it as per machine's instructions.
4. Stir in the cacao nibs before freezing it.
5. Place the cacao ice cream in the freezer for 1 hour.
6. Serve.

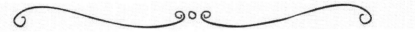

Strawberry Mousse

Prep + Cook time: 10 minutes | Serves: 2

Nutritional Info (per serving)

Calories	Fat (g)	Protein (g)	Carbs (g)	Fiber (g)
385	12	6.1	16.1	0.5

Ingredients:

1 can organic full-fat coconut milk, hardened part only

3 tbs. organic freeze-dried strawberries

2 tbs. organic unrefined granular sweetener

Directions:

1. Put everything into a blender jar.
2. Pulse the ingredients together until smooth.
3. Refrigerate well until chilled.
4. Serve with desired garnish.

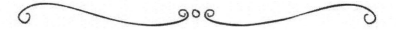

Chocolate Turtles

Prep + Cook time: 10 minutes | Serves: 4

Nutritional Info (per serving)

Calories	Fat (g)	Protein (g)	Carbs (g)	Fiber (g)
332	3.1	7.7	23.2	0.4

Ingredients:

For the caramel mixture:

1 1/2 cups organic medjool dates (pitted)

2 tbs. organic almond butter

2 tbs. water (filtered/purified)

1 tbs. organic coconut oil

1 pinch Himalayan pink salt

For the mix-in:

1 cup organic pecans (chopped)

For the chocolate coating:

1 cup sugar-free mini-chocolate chips

1 tbs. organic coconut oil

Directions:

1. Blend the caramel mixture in a blender jug
2. Fold in the pecans and mix them gently.
3. Pour caramel mixture over a baking sheet lined with a wax paper spoon by spoon.
4. Place them caramel bites in the refrigerator for 30 minutes.
5. Now melt the chocolate chips with coconut oil in a bowl by heating in a microwave for 3 minutes.
6. Dip the caramel bites in the chocolate to coat them well.
7. Return the bites to the refrigerator for 30 minutes.
8. Serve.

Lemon Mousse Tarts
Prep + Cook time: 10 minutes | Serves: 6

Nutritional Info (per serving)

Calories	Fat (g)	Protein (g)	Carbs (g)	Fiber (g)
383	13.1	4.5	9.1	0.3

Ingredients:

For the mousse:

1 can organic full-fat coconut milk

2 tbs. organic lemon juice

2 tbs. granular swerve

For the crust:

1/2 cup organic raw pecans

2 organic medjool dates

1/2 tbs. organic coconut oil

1/8 teaspoon organic vanilla bean powder

1 pinch Himalayan pink salt

Directions:

1. Crush and grind all the ingredients for crust in a food processor.
2. Divide this mixture into a greased muffin tray.
3. Press the mixture firmly in the cups.
4. Refrigerate the crust for 15 minutes.
5. Meanwhile, blend the ingredients for the mousse.
6. Fill the crust with the mousse.
7. Refrigerate for 30 minutes.
8. Serve

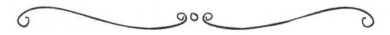

Simple Chocolate Mousse
Prep + Cook time: 10 minutes | Serves: 2

Nutritional Info (per serving)

Calories	Fat (g)	Protein (g)	Carbs (g)	Fiber (g)
215	5	2	13.1	0.2

Ingredients:

1 cup organic full-fat coconut milk

1 tbs. organic raw cacao powder

2 tbs. organic unrefined granular sweetener

Directions:

1. Put everything into a blender jar.
2. Pulse the ingredients together until smooth.
3. Refrigerate well until chilled.
4. Serve with desired garnish.
5. Enjoy.

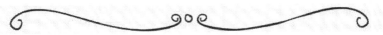

Vanilla Bean Ice Cream
Prep + Cook time: 10 minutes | Serves: 2

Nutritional Info (per serving)

Calories	Fat (g)	Protein (g)	Carbs (g)	Fiber (g)
225	15.2	6.2	32.1	0.4

Ingredients:

2 cups full-fat organic coconut milk

1/2 cup organic granular swerve

2 teaspoons organic vanilla extract	1 teaspoon organic vanilla bean powder
	1 pinch Himalayan pink salt

Directions:

1. Put everything into the blender jug.
2. Blend them together until smooth.
3. Transfer the mixture to an ice maker and churn it as per machine's instructions.
4. Place the vanilla ice cream in the freezer for 1 hour.
5. Serve.

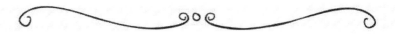

Pumpkin Spice Butter Cups

Prep + Cook time: 10 minutes | Serves: 6

Nutritional Info (per serving)

Calories	*Fat (g)*	*Protein (g)*	*Carbs (g)*	*Fiber (g)*
317	13.5	6	20	0.4

Ingredients:

For the filling:

1/2 cup organic almond butter	2 tbs. organic coconut oil
1/2 cup organic medjool dates (pitted)	1-2 teaspoons organic pumpkin spice
	1 pinch Himalayan pink salt

For the chocolate:

1 cup sugar free minichocolate chips

1 tbs. organic coconut oil

Directions:

1. Put everything for the filling in blender jug.
2. Blend them together until smooth.
3. First, divide the filling in the greased muffin cup of a tray.
4. Refrigerate them for 30 minutes until set.
5. Melt chocolate in a bowl by heating in a microwave.
6. Now divide the chocolate into the refrigerated muffin cups.
7. Refrigerate again for 15 minutes.
8. Serve.

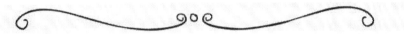

Chocolate Fudge Tarts

Prep + Cook time: 10 minutes | Serves: 4

Nutritional Info (per serving)

Calories	Fat (g)	Protein (g)	Carbs (g)	Fiber (g)
319	10.5	6.7	14.3	1.2

Ingredients:

For the crust:

1 cup organic walnuts

1 tbs. organic coconut oil

1 cup organic medjool dates (pitted)

1 pinch Himalayan pink salt

For the filling:

1/2 cup organic almond butter

1/4 cup organic raw cacao powder

1/2 cup organic coconut oil

1 pinch Himalayan pink salt

1/2 cup organic date nectar

Directions:

1. Crush and grind all the ingredients for crust in a food processor.
2. Divide this mixture into a greased muffin tray.
3. Press the mixture firmly in the cups.
4. Refrigerate the crust for 15 minutes.
5. Meanwhile, blend the ingredients for filling.
6. Fill the crust with the filling.
7. Refrigerate for 30 minutes.
8. Serve

Apple Caramel Bars

Prep + Cook time: 10 minutes | Serves: 6

Nutritional Info (per serving)

Calories	Fat (g)	Protein (g)	Carbs (g)	Fiber (g)
372	12	9.8	21.7	1.5

Ingredients:

For the crust:

1 cup almond flour

1 tbs. organic coconut flour

1/4 cup organic date nectar

1/8 teaspoon organic vanilla bean powder

1/4 cup organic coconut oil

1 pinch Himalayan pink salt

For the filling:

4 small organic apples

1 cup organic medjool dates (pitted)

2 tbs. organic coconut oil

1 teaspoon organic lemon juice (freshly squeezed)

1/8 teaspoon organic vanilla bean powder

1/4 teaspoon organic ground cinnamon

1 pinch Himalayan pink salt

For the topping:

1/2 cup organic almond butter

1/2 cup organic coconut oil

1/2 cup organic date nectar

1/2 teaspoon organic vanilla bean powder

1/8 teaspoon Himalayan pink salt

Directions:

1. Combine every ingredient for the crust in a bowl.
2. Spread this mixture in an 8x8 inch baking dish.
3. Put all the ingredients for filling in a food processor and pulse until finely chopped.
4. Transfer the filling over the crust over the filling.
5. Whisk the ingredients for topping and cover the filling with it.
6. Place the filled dish in the refrigerator for 30 minutes.
7. Serve.

Pistachio Fudge with Sea Salt
Prep + Cook time: 10 minutes | Serves: 6

Nutritional Info (per serving)

Calories	Fat (g)	Protein (g)	Carbs (g)	Fiber (g)
264	7.1	2.7	17	0.5

Ingredients:

For the fudge:

1 cup organic pistachios (chopped and/or whole)

1 cup organic coconut oil (melted/liquid)

1/4 cup organic raw cacao powder

1/4 cup organic date nectar

1/4 cup organic almond butter

1 teaspoon organic vanilla bean powder

For the topping:

sea salt

Directions:

1. Put everything for the fudge in a bowl and mix them well.
2. Divide the mixture into 24 muffin cups.
3. Place the muffin cups in the refrigerator for 10 minutes.
4. Sprinkle sea salt on top of them.
5. Return them to the refrigerator for 1 hour.
6. Serve.

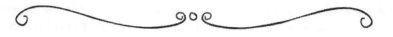

Chocolate Cauliflower Cream Bowl
Prep + Cook time: 10 minutes | Serves: 4

Calories	Fat (g)	Protein (g)	Carbs (g)	Fiber (g)
366	6.4	8.7	21.3	1.1

Ingredients:

Cream:

1 large organic frozen banana

1 cup of organic frozen cauliflower rice

1/4 cup + 1 tbs. almond milk

2 tbs. organic raw cacao powder

1 tbs. organic almond butter

For the toppings:

1/2 cup organic wild blueberries

1-2 tbs. organic raw cacao nibs

Directions:

1. Put everything into a blender jug.
2. Blend well until smooth.
3. Garnish with the desired toppings.
4. Refrigerate well.
5. Serve.

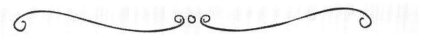

Chocolate Avocado Pistachio Truffles
Prep + Cook time: 10 minutes | Serves: 6

Nutritional Info (per serving)

Calories	Fat (g)	Protein (g)	Carbs (g)	Fiber (g)
295	3.9	3.3	36.2	1.5

Ingredients:

For the truffles:

1 organic avocado

1 tbs. organic coconut oil

1 cup organic medjool dates

1 tbs. filtered/purified water

1/2 cup organic almond butter

1/8 teaspoon organic vanilla bean powder

2 tbs. organic raw cacao powder

1 pinch Himalayan pink salt

For the add-in:

1/4 cup organic pistachios (chopped)

For the coating:

1/4 cup organic pistachios (ground)

Directions:

1. Grind all the ingredients for truffles in a food processor
2. Fold in the chopped pistachios and mix well.
3. Use wet hands to prepare small balls out of this mixture.
4. Roll these balls in the pistachio ground then place them in a baking sheet.
5. Refrigerate for 15 minutes.
6. Serve.

Chocolate Avocado Frosting

Prep + Cook time: 10 minutes | Serves: 4

Nutritional Info (per serving)

Calories	*Fat (g)*	*Protein (g)*	*Carbs (g)*	*Fiber (g)*
315	9	1.4	21.7	0.4

Ingredients:

2 organic avocados

1/4 cup organic raw cacao powder

1/4 cup organic almond butter

1/4 cup organic date nectar

1 - 2 pinches Himalayan pink salt

Directions:

1. Put everything into a blender.
2. Blend them well together until smooth.
3. Refrigerate until chilled.
4. Serve.

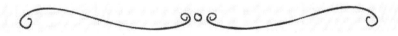

Tahini Brownie Truffles
Prep + Cook time: 10 minutes | Serves: 6

Nutritional Info (per serving)

Calories	*Fat (g)*	*Protein (g)*	*Carbs (g)*	*Fiber (g)*
386	8.9	3.1	11.9	1.3

Ingredients:

For the truffles:

1 cup organic medjool dates (pitted)	2 tbs. homemade almond milk
1/2 cup organic tahini	1/2 teaspoon organic vanilla bean powder
1/2 cup almond flour	
1/4 cup organic raw cacao powder	1 pinch Himalayan pink salt

For the coating:

1/4 cup organic raw cacao powder

1/4 cup organic date nectar

1/4 cup organic coconut oil

For the topping:

1/4 cup organic walnuts (chopped)

Directions:

1. Put everything for the truffles in a food processor.
2. Grind everything together and make small balls out of it.
3. Place these balls in a baking sheet lined with wax paper.
4. Mix the cocoa powder with coconut oil and date nectar.
5. Roll the balls in this mixture to coat them well.
6. Now coat each ball with chopped walnuts.
7. Place them in the baking sheet again.
8. Refrigerate for 15 minutes.
9. Serve.

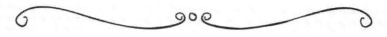

Almond Fudge Cups
Prep + Cook time: 10 minutes | Serves: 6

Nutritional Info (per serving)

Calories	Fat (g)	Protein (g)	Carbs (g)	Fiber (g)
383	13.2	3.7	37.8	1.2

Ingredients:

For the fudge:

1 cup almonds, chopped

1 cup organic coconut oil, melted

1/4 cup organic raw cacao powder

1/4 cup organic date nectar

1/4 cup organic almond butter

1 teaspoon organic vanilla bean powder

For the topping:

sea salt

Directions:

1. Put everything for almond fudge cup in a bowl and mix them well.
2. Divide the mixture into 24 muffin cups.
3. Place the muffin cups in the refrigerator for 10 minutes.
4. Sprinkle sea salt on top of them.
5. Return them to the refrigerator for 1 hour.
6. Serve.

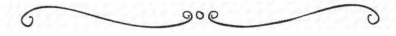

Forest Chia Seed Pudding

Prep + Cook time: 10 minutes | Serves: 2

Nutritional Info (per serving)

Calories	Fat (g)	Protein (g)	Carbs (g)	Fiber (g)
377	11.2	6.1	12	0.2

Ingredients:

For the chia pudding:

2 cups homemade almond milk

1/2 cup organic chia seeds

2 tbs. organic unrefined granular sweetener

For the dark cherry chia jam:

2 cups of organic dark cherries (pitted)

2 tbs. organic chia seeds

2 tbs. filtered/purified water

1 tbs. organic lemon juice (freshly squeezed)

For the chocolate add-in:

1/4 cup sugar free minichocolate chips

1 teaspoon organic coconut oil

For the dark cherry add-in:

1 cup organic dark cherries (pitted)

Directions:

1. Put everything for chia pudding in a blender.
2. Blend them together for 30 seconds without breaking the chia seeds.
3. Pour the pudding in a bowl and refrigerate it for 15 minutes.

4. Blende the chia jam mixture in a blender for 30 seconds.
5. Melt the chocolate chipswith coconut oil in a bowl by heating in the microwave.
6. Add layers of chia pudding, chia jam, chocolate and cherries in the serving glasses.
7. Refrigerate for 30 minutes before serving.
8. Enjoy.

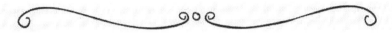

Dragon Fruit Chia Pudding

Prep + Cook time: 10 minutes | Serves: 2

Nutritional Info (per serving)

Calories	*Fat (g)*	*Protein (g)*	*Carbs (g)*	*Fiber (g)*
248	4	7.6	11	0.4

Ingredients:

For the chia pudding:

2 cups homemade almond milk

1/2 cup organic chia seeds

1 teaspoon organic vanilla extract

For the dragon fruit layer:

1 packet frozen organic pitaya (dragon fruit)

1 organic banana

Directions:

1. Put everything for chia pudding in a blender.

2. Blend them together for 30 seconds without breaking the chia seeds.
3. Pour the pudding in a bowl and refrigerate it for 15 minutes.
4. Blend the dragon fruits layer ingredients in a blender for 30 seconds.
5. Add layers of chia pudding, and dragon fruit layer in the serving glasses.
6. Refrigerate for 30 minutes before serving.
7. Enjoy.

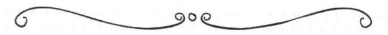

Black Forest Bars
Prep + Cook time: 10 minutes | Serves: 6

Nutritional Info (per serving)

Calories	*Fat (g)*	*Protein (g)*	*Carbs (g)*	*Fiber (g)*
227	6.5	7.2	35.4	0.3

Ingredients:

For the brownie base:

1 cup organic walnuts

4 organic medjool dates (pitted)

1/4 cup organic raw cacao powder

2 tbs. organic refined coconut oil

1 pinch Himalayan pink salt

For the cherry filling:

1 1/2 cups of organic cherries (pitted, halved)

8 organic medjool dates (pitted)

1 tbs. organic refined coconut oil

For the chocolate topping:

1 organic avocado

2 tbs. organic date nectar

2 tbs organic coconut oil

2 tbs. organic almond butter

2 tbs. organic raw cacao powder

Directions:

1. Put everything for the crust in the food processor.
2. Grind this mixture until crumbly.
3. Spread the crust mixture in a greased baking pan and press it firmly.
4. Gently blend the filling ingredients for few seconds in a blender.
5. Transfer the filling into the crust.
6. Blend the topping ingredients in the blender.
7. Spread the topping over the filling.
8. Refrigerate for 30 minutes until it is set.
9. Slice and serve.

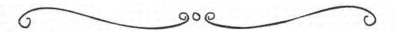

Cranberry Lemon Ball Truffles

Prep + Cook time: 10 minutes | Serves: 6

Nutritional Info (per serving)

Calories	Fat (g)	Protein (g)	Carbs (g)	Fiber (g)
223	6.5	1.6	17.8	0.3

Ingredients:

For the balls:

1 1/2 cups almond flour

1/4 cup organic lemon juice

1/4 cup organic coconut oil

1/4 cup organic erythritol syrup

1/3 cup organic coconut flour

1 tbs. organic lemon zest

1/2 teaspoon organic pure vanilla extract

1-2 pinches Himalayan salt

For the add-in:

1/4 cup organic dried cranberries

Directions:

1. Combine all the ingredients for the balls in a blender.
2. Fold in the cranberries then make small balls out of it.
3. Refrigerate the balls for 30 minutes.
4. Serve.

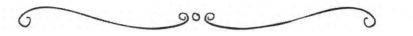

Cacao Almond Balls
Prep + Cook time: 10 minutes | Serves: 6

Nutritional Info (per serving)

Calories	*Fat (g)*	*Protein (g)*	*Carbs (g)*	*Fiber (g)*
311	4.8	3.6	18.2	0.1

Ingredients:

1 cup of organic raw almonds

1/2 cup organic almond butter

1/4 cup almond flour

1/4 cup organic raw cacao powder

2 tbs. organic hemp oil

2 tbs. organic maca powder

1 tbs. organic date nectar

1/2 teaspoon organic vanilla bean powder

Directions:

1. Toss all the ingredients to a processor until it forms a thick paste.
2. Make small balls using a spoon and place them cover a baking sheet.
3. Refrigerate it for 30 minutes.
4. Serve.

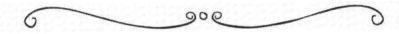

Blueberry Protein Energy Balls
Prep + Cook time: 10 minutes | Serves: 6

Nutritional Info (per serving)

Calories	Fat (g)	Protein (g)	Carbs (g)	Fiber (g)
321	2.7	4,1	14,1	0.5

Ingredients:

1 cup organic dried blueberries

1 cup organic medjool dates (pitted)

2 tbs. Yuva' Vanilla Vegan Protein Powder*

1 tbs. organic almond butter

1 teaspoon organic vanilla bean powder

Directions:

1. Toss all the ingredients to a processor until it forms a thick paste.
2. Make small balls using a spoon and place them cover a baking sheet.
3. Refrigerate it for 30 minutes.
4. Serve.

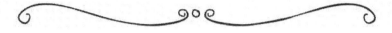

Chocolate Avocado Ice Cream with Almond Butter
Prep + Cook time: 10 minutes | Serves: 2

Nutritional Info (per serving)

Calories	Fat (g)	Protein (g)	Carbs (g)	Fiber (g)
166	8.7	2	21.2	0.2

Ingredients

Ice cream:

1 can organic full-fat coconut milk

1/4 cup organic raw cacao powder

2 organic avocados (pitted)

1/4 - 1/2 cup xylitol

For the swirl:

1/2 cup organic almond butter

1 tbs. organic date nectar

Directions:

1. Blend the avocado ice cream ingredients in a blender jug.

2. Mix almond butter with date nectar.
3. Top the ice cream with butter mixture.
4. Refrigerate for 1 hour.
5. Garnish with coconut flakes.
6. Serve

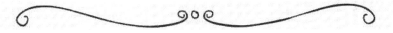

Raspberry and Chocolate Ice Cream Squares
Prep + Cook time: 10 minutes | Serves: 6

Nutritional Info (per serving)

Calories	*Fat (g)*	*Protein (g)*	*Carbs (g)*	*Fiber (g)*
227	0.5	0.9g	51.4g	0.1g

Ingredients:

For the ice cream:

2 organic avocados (pitted)	1/4 cup organic date nectar
1 can organic full-fat coconut milk	1/4 teaspoon organic vanilla bean powder
1/2 cup organic raw cacao powder	1/4 teaspoon Himalayan pink salt

For the add-in:

1 cup organic freeze-dried raspberries

For the topping:

1/2 cup organic freeze-dried raspberries

Directions:

7. Blend the ingredients for ice cream in a blender jug.

8. Fold in the raspberries and spread the mixture in a baking pan.
9. Top it with raspberries.
10. Refrigerate for 1 hour.
11. Slice and serve.

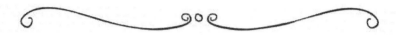

Avocado Ice Cream Bars

Prep + Cook time: 10 minutes | Serves: 6

Nutritional Info (per serving)

Calories	Fat (g)	Protein (g)	Carbs (g)	Fiber (g)
213	1.5	1.2	53.2	0.5

Ingredients:

1/2 cup strawberries

1 can organic full-fat coconut milk

2 organic avocados (pitted)

1/4 cup organic date nectar

1/4 teaspoon organic vanilla bean powder

1/4 teaspoon Himalayan pink salt

½ cup strawberry slices for topping

Directions:

1. Blend the ingredients for ice cream in a blender jug.
2. Spread the mixture in a baking pan.
3. Top it with strawberry slices.
4. Refrigerate for 1 hour.

Slice into bars and serve.

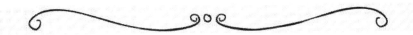

Conclusion:

Lectins are mostly present in the seeds of the plants and are considered to be harmful. There is also a considerable amount of research supporting the role of plant foods in our body despite the fact that they are considered harmful. According to varying types of the plants the lectins levels may vary from plant to plant. The research that has been on lentils have mostly been performed on the animals and test tube studies. Lectins have been credited with the many medical complications and the diseases like inflammation and digestion issues despite of the fact that researchers have focused on a specific lectin rather than the plants carrying it as a whole.

It is, however, at this stage, hard to completely assign lectins as useless. Certain studies have shown them to beneficial in smaller quantities to help the digestive system and help remove bacteria. However, more research needs to be done on this. As described, certain recipes can be made to have lectin free diet and meal prepping will assist in this activity. It is important that we start taking our health and things we consume on daily basis seriously. Check the nutritional values of each food we cook to avoid diseases in the long-run.

15201722R00204

Printed in Germany
by Amazon Distribution
GmbH, Leipzig